Dental
Success Stories

25 inspirational true stories from the experts in dentistry

Nafisa Mughal and
Dr Shakir Mughal

First printing: 2018
ISBN-13: 978-1726012058
ISBN-10: 1726012050

British Cataloguing Publication Data: A catalogue record of this book is available from The British Library.

Also available on Kindle.

Charity

'We make a living by what we get ... but we make a life
by what we give.'
Winston Churchill

We are proud to say that for each book sold, we will be donating £1 to a charity in India called Food For Life Vrindavan (FFLV). As parents of a beautiful daughter, we could not help but get involved as soon as we heard what this charity stands for and does.

FFLV has been working in Vrindavan, India since 1991. The charity aims to educate girls living in poverty, empowering them to transform their lives and communities. The three FFLV schools provide free education, meals, clean water and medical help to over 1500 girls whose lives would otherwise be ones of poverty and lack. FFLV also works with the girls' families and community towards a range of outcomes.

Child marriage and child abuse often occur when girls are born into poor families in India. Girls are seen as a further economic burden on households that are already poverty stricken. By providing free education and nutritious meals to these girls, they improve their physical health, mental wellbeing and, ultimately, they have better lives.

If you would like further information about this charity or would like to make a donation, please visit www.fflv.org.

Contents

Introduction

This book contains twenty-five stories from some of the top experts in the dental world, told in their own words. Every story is in the expert's own voice and showcases their individual journey, how they got to where they are. Not only have the experts provided us with their stories, they have also provided us with some incredible tips for success.

We have purposefully chosen experts from all parts of dentistry, including dental hygienists, dental coaches, specialists, academics, general dental practitioners, business owners and individuals who have left clinical dentistry and built a new career.

We hope you not only enjoy reading these stories but also feel inspired by them and apply the tips to transform your own life!

'By changing nothing, nothing changes.'
Tony Robbins

We want to stress that we are not preaching that to be successful you must be an expert or be well known in the industry. We merely chose well-known individuals so the reader could easily relate to them.

Why we wrote this book

Our profession currently stands at a juxtaposition. On the one hand, the technology and materials available currently in dentistry allow the profession to provide the highest standard of care and more advanced treatments to more of the population. On the other hand, there seems to be a general level of gloom and doom within the profession from increasing litigation, pressures from NHS dentistry, rising business expenses and overheads, uncertainties with the future of NHS dentistry, lack of confidence in newly qualified graduates and what seems like more and more red tape each year!

With all of this going on we wanted to try to make a difference within the profession and came up with the idea of this book of stories to inspire our profession.

What is success?

This question will be answered by our experts as within each story our experts have given us their own definition of success and what it means to them.

Is success important?

Since you are reading this book we hope and assume that success is important to you. In the dental profession we have all achieved a great level of success already through our education and qualifications. What matters next is how you use this success and build upon it to create the future you deserve. Without striving for success, you will have no real vision, goal or purpose for life.

How to read this book

You can read this book in whichever manner you like but please ensure you read our final chapter, The Secret to Dental Success as it is here where we have combined all the top tips from our experts into a list of success principles. You may already be familiar with some or all of the principles but take a minute to think if you are actually applying them.

'The principles always work if you work the principles.'
Jack Canfield

Try not to rush through the book; take your time and try to get out as much as you can from each story you read. Some stories will speak louder to you than others and some will have more meaning than others. This book represents a culmination of over 200 years of experience, all ready and waiting for you!

You Don't Yet Know What You Don't Yet Know

Dr Raj Ahlowalia
BDS LDSRCSEn

Dr Raj Ahlowalia graduated from Guy's Hospital in 1991 and since then has pursued a journey of continuing education, studying with, and then teaching alongside, some of the finest dentists in the world. Between 2006 and 2007, Dr Ahlowalia also featured in two seasons of the *Extreme Makeover UK* television show. Dr Ahlowalia now divides his time between treating patients at his private practice in Bedfordshire and teaching colleagues comprehensive dentistry, which involves techniques blended from his years at The Pankey and Spear Institutes.

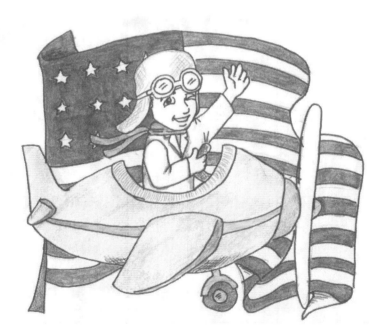

Dentistry was not a childhood dream for me. All I ever wanted to do as a child was become an airline pilot but ultimately my eyesight let me down. It was my form tutor at school who persuaded me to apply to university. Being a bit of a nerd and technology geek, I initially applied for both astrophysics and dental schools. However, it was my dad who brought reality home to me in typically Asian parent fashion by saying: "Go be a dentist. Do you really think NASA needs an Indian boy from the London 'burbs?!"

That sage advice led to my ultimate graduation from Guy's Hospital in 1991 with a shiny dental degree and soon after I completed my VT training year at a practice in rural Bedfordshire. 1991 was a time of great upheaval within the profession, as a new NHS contract was looming. I recall looking at the contract with my boss at the time and wondering how we could deliver high quality dentistry under the proposed new system.

By the time the new NHS contract began in April 1995, we decided with much difficulty to leave the NHS system and become an independent private practice, setting reasonable fees and providing simple treatment plans.

By the early 2000s, things were settled at the practice, our 'formula' having been generally accepted by our patients. However, personally I felt I needed to be offering something more as a 'private' dentist.

A close friend and colleague at the time persuaded me to attend a one-day seminar with a 'big name' American cosmetic dentist who was coming to present in London. After a little arguing over the extortionate £100 fee but appeasement via the promise of a home-made curry at his mum's, I received my first glimpse of a standard of dentistry I had never before dreamed of, let alone been taught. In enquiring of the speaker where we could begin to learn this level of dentistry we were advised to head to the US, not only to study the principles of cosmetic dentistry but also how to marry that with stable function for long term predictability.

We agreed to build our knowledge together; my friend would go to The Pankey Institute in Florida to study functional dentistry, whilst I would learn American-style cosmetic dentistry in New York.

Soon after, my new-found skills landed me a role on the *Extreme Makeover UK* television show. It was during this time that I rapidly recognised the big holes in my knowledge of dentistry for complex cases, which often had to be finished by my friend. I recognised the need to build stability into such cases from the design stage rather than at the end. So I headed to the Pankey Institute to begin my own journey through their continuum.

It was within my first hour at the institute that I learnt the single most important lesson of my educational pathway. "You don't yet know what you don't yet know," whispered Dr Steve Ratcliff, my lecturer that morning, my mentor and now dear friend. Along with the rest of the faculty he taught me what The Pankey Institute called 'Comprehensive Dentistry'. It was a way of understanding how all the dental disciplines interconnect. That year of travelling back and forth to the institute for seven separate weeks of learning completely transformed my dentistry.

The knowledge I gained from the institute allowed me to choose to become either an interdisciplinary or multidisciplinary dentist, depending on whether I wished to perform all the specialities myself or work within a team. I chose to expand my knowledge further and educate myself in as many of the specialities as I could at the same time. My journey took me around the world, through Europe, the US and South America, learning everything from orthodontics, implantology, periodontology and bone grafting to hypnotherapy, neuro-linguistic programming (NLP) and psychology.

By now I was teaching and mentoring regularly in Europe, Arizona and Florida. However, in my dental practice I had come full circle. In the very same room in which I started my career as an NHS VT, I continue to practise as a general dentist, only now with the benefit of several lifetimes of learning, knowledge and expertise passed on by caring mentors, colleagues and friends.

Finally, and most importantly, it was my VT trainer Dr Robin Varma, who for over two decades worked in a room not two metres from mine, who taught me the most about being a good dentist. Irrespective of all the courses I attended and knowledge I gained, Robin taught me more than just the art of being a practitioner or running a business but how to truly care for people, more than any dental school, dental book or course ever could, and I thank him for that. Robin did it all naturally. I'm still working on it!

What is success?

I suppose I see success as a measure of personal happiness and the ability to sleep at night, stress free. For some that will be because bills are paid, there's money in the bank and something to spare for whatever luxuries make us smile. For others it will be that family are provided for, and that they have smiles on their faces. And for some it will be the validation that comes through recognition of our abilities and work; the smiles we put on the faces of our patients.

For me it is a little sprinkling of each and the happiness of my staff and those who I am charged with caring for and the relationships I have built with them over my career.

Top tips for success

Recognise in every human being you meet another person just like you; a person who loves and laughs, who feels hurt and pain just like you do. The day we appreciate everyone else as an equally valid human being will be the day our relationship with each individual we meet grows and blossoms. With that comes a certain joy that the self-absorbed will never truly appreciate.

Take time to connect with people. It brings rewards mere money can never buy.

The Yes Factor

Mhari Coxon
RDH

Mhari Coxon is a renowned dental hygienist. She qualified at King's College in 1996 and since then has paved the way for hygienists not only to grow and become outstanding practitioners, but to realise that dental hygiene is not a one stop career. Mhari is seen as an inspirational figure in the dental community and has now branched out in the world of marketing.

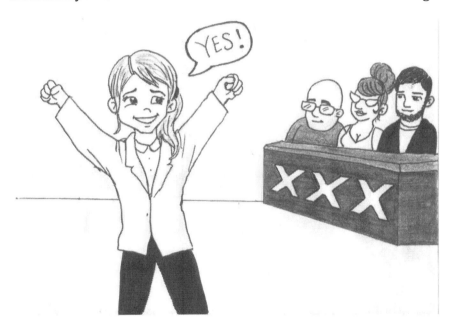

For me, getting into dentistry was a happy accident. I think dentists choose dentistry whereas I feel I didn't choose dentistry, it chose me!

I remember I was killing time during the summer holidays and landed a job as a dental nurse. I was set to go off and do business studies but actually quite enjoyed dental nursing, so I decided to stay on and complete a dental nursing course in the evenings, up in Glasgow, in which I qualified in 1994.

I then moved to London at age 18 and became an oral health educator in an anaesthetic clinic. I found this difficult as I was educating parents whose children's teeth were already coming out. This motivated me to become a hygienist as I felt I wasn't making the difference in people's lives that I wanted to.

I managed to get into King's College on my first try but decided to defer for a year and go travelling in Malaysia. I feel this was so important in my journey as it got me used to living within a multicultural society.

After returning from Malaysia and subsequently completing my hygienist training in 1996, I decided to stay on as a staff hygienist and later became a clinical tutor.

I continued teaching when I had my three children. Dental hygiene is a great career to work around being a mum; I found it very flexible and it fitted into my life as a parent.

However, as much as I loved teaching, I couldn't keep it up for very long. It was poorly paid and by the time I had paid for childcare, I barely broke even. I saw it as my 'charity' day and eventually, with a heavy heart, I had to give it up.

In 2002 I sadly lost my mother as well as having my son diagnosed with autism. That was a dark and horrible year, but I vowed I would not let it beat me.

In 2005 I left King's College and started working at the Fresh Breath Clinic. The dentist there owned Dentyl pH mouthwash and invited me to speak about a new flavour. It was my first time speaking in public and the first time I had challenged myself to learn new things. I was so nervous, standing up there in front of 600 people, holding onto the lectern for grim death! I relaxed after I told a joke that made the audience roar with laughter – and made me relax and enjoy it! I walked away from the lecture feeling like I was in my element, and that was just me, what I was meant to be doing.

Through this, I met Tracy Posner, who worked at Positive Communications. She encouraged me to do more speaking. She was a key catalyst for a lot of my career. Her passion and support and belief were such fuel. She gave me the opportunity to lecture, and the opportunity to move in to business management and post graduate education.

At this point I just said yes to everything and worked out how I would do it afterwards!

I extended my knowledge of non-surgical periodontics by doing some post graduate training at the Eastman in 2006 and realised that you don't learn everything at university, even though you think you know a lot! It was after that that I put myself forward for the hygienist awards, and fortunately won that title.

That was a wow moment! I realised if people thought I was good enough to win, I had to live up to that standard. It changed the way I worked and made me push myself more.

I began writing articles and was asked to do more speaking as well as working in practice. It was starting to become a bit of a juggling act. I found that the more you say yes to doing, the more offers you get to do things! I guess this is where the adage comes from of asking a busy person to do something and you'll know it'll get done.

Later in 2008, as I was still juggling more and more speaking and writing roles, it was announced that CPD would become compulsory for DCPs. I teamed up with a friend of mine who was actually my tutor at King's, Joanna Jones, to create CPD for DCPs.

I hadn't a clue how to run a business but just went for it. I think in this case ignorance was bliss as we made it work!

In 2010, GSK asked me to speak for them about the gum smart kit, the chief aim of which was to empower patients to ask about their gum health. The kit was so amazing, it won an award! At the same time, I found it to be such a positive experience that it made me feel ready to step into the world of marketing. I didn't realise that marketing had a name; it was what I loved doing and I wanted to do more of it.

In 2011 I was shocked to be voted number 15 in the dentistry top 50. It was like girl power as a lot of hygienists and nurses were voting for me! I didn't think I deserved it but again, it spurred me on to prove my worth. In 2010 I came in at number 5.

All this juggling soon started to take its toll on my clinical work as I was away from clinic more and more. My patients were starting to feel upset about this and soon I had to make a decision; either stay and work in surgery all the time or leave. I decided to leave.

I was then approached by Philips and decided to work for them. Soon after, the laws for tooth whitening changed. In 2012, I invited all the major companies that offered whitening to collaborate to raise awareness for patients. This was the start of the Tooth Whitening Information Group, which is now run by the Oral Health Foundation. It's the achievement I am most proud of during my time at Philips.

After five years with Philips, I decided I needed a new challenge. The work had become repetitive and there was no room to grow or move to a more senior role.

As I was redundant and out of work I decided to start my master's in marketing at Liverpool University. I gained the honour of Outstanding Contribution to Dental Hygiene and Therapy as well as becoming a trustee of the Oral Health Foundation in 2015 and realised that I was done in dentistry. I wanted to leave while I was at the top of my game!

I moved out of dentistry and began working on other projects. I was feeling the joy of marketing, as I felt I was doing it for the right reasons, helping others as part of my job!

I left that role in 2016 to join GSK in my current role as global marketing manager in oral health and skin health, and I absolutely love it! I would actively encourage people to have two or even more careers, and not to be frightened to step away.

I feel that I have had a fantastic 20 years in dentistry and am now aiming to reach the same level within marketing.

What is success?

I will tell you when I get there, but I have had some great moments!

For me, you can only be successful if you are continuing to grow and learn. Learning is a lifelong activity; you don't simply stop when you think you know it all because in fact, you will never know it all.

Coming out of your comfort zone and having that 'washing machine' feeling in your stomach means that something good is going to happen if you just push through it.

For me to be a success, I wish to leave the world in a better condition than when I came into it, and when I go I want to be remembered as someone who actually made a difference.

Top tips for success

Be engaged and be curious. Ask people why something is rather than just taking a back seat.

When someone asks you to do something, just say yes! Figure out the logistics afterwards. Even if you don't have the answers straight away, you can find someone who does. Never be frightened of failing. As clinicians we find failure very difficult but often failure leads to growth, and we must keep growing.

The Writer

Dr Len D'Cruz
BDS LDSRCS MFGDP(UK) LLM PGC MedEd Dip FOd

Dr Len D'Cruz graduated in 1990 from the Royal London Hospital. He is a past chairman of the BDA Young Dentist Committee and examiner for the Faculty of General Dental Practitioners. He is currently a member of the BDA General Dental Practitioners Committee and a non-executive director of the BDA elected to the Principal Executive Committee. Len divides his time between his work for Dental Protection and his own general practice where he is a vocational trainer for the London Deanery. He is a dental tutor in the Eastern Deanery and a lecturer on the MA Dental Law and Ethics course at the University of Bedfordshire.

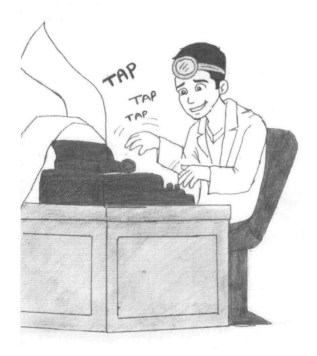

I always had a real passion for sciences at school but also writing and studying English. During my A-levels I was contemplating studying either English or dentistry at university. Bizarrely, it was my English teacher who persuaded me to choose dentistry! She told me I could always come back to writing in the future, which, prophetically, is what happened.

After spending a great five years at the Royal London I decided to do vocational training (VT), despite it not being mandatory at that time. The principal owned three practices including one in Woodford; I worked at all three practices during my vocational training year.

At the end of my VT year, I decided I really wanted to write about my experience of vocational training. As it happened, the editor of the British Dental Journal (BDJ), Margaret Seward, had been my oral surgery tutor and she gave me the opportunity to write a series of three articles. This was my first major writing accomplishment and gave birth to my writing career! The swelling pride of seeing your name in print has never really gone away, particularly when it is in a peer-reviewed publication.

A couple of years following VT, I was given the opportunity to purchase the Woodford practice from my previous VT trainer. I continue to still work and run the Woodford practice alongside my wife. We have grown the practice from a 1.5 to a 7-surgery practice.

My passion for writing provided me with a parallel career alongside clinical dentistry. I began to write more articles for the BDJ and The Probe as well as The Dentist. Writing letters to the BDJ on specific issues fostered my belief that you could contribute to patient care as much with your pen as with your drill. During these times there was no social media or internet so to become known meant getting myself out there and involving myself with all the big organisations, including the British Dental Association (BDA), and Faculty of General Dental Practitioners (FGDP).

Due to my writing, my involvement with the FGDP, and my role in setting up the BDA Young Dentist Committee, I was approached by Dental Protection in 1997 to become their youngest dento-legal adviser ever appointed. Soon after I also became the youngest examiner for the FGDP, examining for the DGDP as it was then before it morphed eventually into the MJDF exam.

During my time at Dental Protection I became very interested in law and decided to do a law degree. In 2005 I completed a master's degree in medical law at Cardiff University. Whilst being a very interesting course, it was not all that relevant to dentistry.

Soon after, I approached Dental Update, keen to write some articles on dental law and ethics. To my surprise the editor, Professor Trevor Burke, told me not to bother with the articles but instead to write a book! After a couple of years of balancing work and a young family, writing in early morning stints, I managed to complete the book, *Legal Aspects of General Dental Practice*, which was published in 2006 by Elsevier. I am now working on the second edition, which should be published soon.

Having listened to Claire Morris, who ran the PG Cert in Dental Education, at a conference I had the idea of setting up a law and ethics course specific to dentistry. I approached Claire at the University of Bedfordshire. She was quite keen to develop more courses for dentists and eventually, over a period of a few years, we managed to develop and launch a recognised degree in Dental Law and Ethics which continues to increase in popularity and now has become a master's degree.

Currently I spend my working week between my practice in Woodford where I'm still enjoying clinical dentistry, working with DPL, and lecturing and teaching on the master's Dental Law and Ethics course at the University of Bedfordshire. I'm also involved with other issues such as NHS regulations and sit on senior BDA committees.

What is success?

For me, success is managing to get a good work life balance whilst making a difference to people's lives, in a good way.

Top tips for success

Say yes to every opportunity you are given and do it well. Over a period of time this will lead to success.

If you have a passion around dentistry, follow that passion.
Be involved in your profession and find a mentor or role model who

will guide your path and inspire you.

Build trust between yourself and the patient by having empathy, being honest, and developing great communication skills – including learning the art of conversation.

The Godfather

Dr Mervyn Druian
BDS (Rand), DGDP (RCS)

Dr Mervyn Druian qualified in Johannesburg in 1969. Mervyn's impact on UK cosmetic dentistry is undeniable. Over a career spanning nearly 50 years, Mervyn has often been heralded as the Godfather of UK cosmetic dentistry – bringing the acclaimed Aesthetic Advantage Programme to the UK as well as running the highly successful London Centre for Cosmetic Dentistry whilst offering his time to philanthropic pursuits. Mervyn is also the past international president of the Alpha Omega Dental Society, a regular contributor to numerous dental journals and a speaker at educational events.

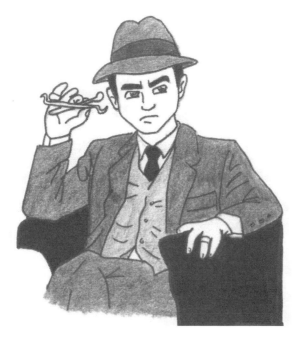

My story begins in Johannesburg. I was lucky enough to obtain my dental degree at one of the top-rated dental universities in the world, at that time. The teaching and technology were light years ahead of anything in the UK.

After qualifying in 1969, I came to the UK to work for two years in the National Health Service (NHS). It was at this time I became a dental course junkie! I went on every course going, regardless of the topic. I also went on some courses in the US, where I met some fantastic people and top speakers.

Following this, I returned to South Africa as I had to complete a mandatory one-year army placement, working as a dentist. This was a fantastic experience as we had complete free range in the army so I could practise everything I had learnt on all those courses!

In about 1974 I decided to set up a practice in Cape Town. It was at this time I met Dr Omer Reed, the father of preventative dentistry and practice management. He came to South Africa to lecture on practice management. As a junior member of the South African Dental Association, I was given the honour of looking after Dr Reed and his wife during their visit. I had never met a guy like him before; he was truly inspirational and doing things in dentistry that were ground breaking. Omer Reed fuelled my passion for dentistry further, and to this day I still love my work and think of it more as a hobby than a job.

After a few years, my family and I came to the realisation that the political situation in South Africa was becoming bleak. We didn't see a long-term future for us there so we emigrated to England. I took associate jobs in Luton and Hampstead, working in the NHS, and we settled into a more peaceful life. It was at this time I started to become more involved in organised dentistry, and I joined the British Dental Association (BDA) and at that time the metropolitan branch of the BDA, becoming secretary and eventually president of the branch.

Being involved in organised dentistry gave me the opportunity to see what was going on in the broader world of UK dentistry at a time when a lot of changes were happening in the NHS. It also allowed me to bring in speakers to lecture at the BDA, including my mentor, Omer Reed, who was encouraging us to leave the NHS and go private, to provide a better level of service for patients. At the time I was the secretary and Laurence Landau was the president. We both decided to work together and encourage dentists to go down the private route. We called it 'independent dentistry' rather than 'private' as in those times, private dentistry was associated with being ripped off! We ended up touring the UK and giving dentists the inspiration and skills to go down the independent route. The BDA took note of what we had achieved and set up the Private Practitioners' Group; at the same time FMC set up a journal called *Independent Dentistry*, now *Private Dentistry*.

Following this, I carried on working in practice, still attended lots of courses, and spent a lot of time with Omer Reed, including annual visits to Phoenix, where he was based.

In 1986, I purchased a very run down mixed dental practice in Belsize Park with a vision to create a high-end private practice. The previous owner was not very ethical; he took all the staff, all the good equipment and all the private patients to his other practice! He left me with a shell of a practice and I had to start from the beginning with a small nucleus of patients. I slowly built up the practice but then in 1988 I had to move location as my lease was not renewed. At this point I joined forces with Ken Spektor, who I knew from dental school. We relocated to new premises in Belsize Park and have been partners ever since.

Omer Reed also became a consultant to our practice and over time, our practice became a model of what Omer had taught us, including the most important part: everything must focus around the customer. The practice thrived and became very profitable and continues to do well. We then began to look at what the next big thing in dentistry would be. At that point aesthetic dentistry was becoming important, as well as implants and bad breath.

I didn't want to go down the road of implants as in the late eighties there were still a lot of complications and failures associated with them. Omer introduced us to a product called Ultradex, which was a treatment modality we began to use heavily in our practice to eradicate bad breath. We became the first practice in the UK to focus on bad breath; we set up a bad breath clinic, treating it with a mixture of Ultradex and intensive hygiene/periodontal treatments. The increase in hygienist treatments made a big impact on the profitability of our practice. It was also in the late eighties that Bob Gibson came to the UK and started talking about veneers, which we incorporated into our practice immediately and enjoyed doing them.

In the nineties, I went to a Chicago dental meeting where I met Larry Rosenthal, whose work was outstanding. I went to his amazing programme in the US and it opened me up to a completely new world. What I learnt became a massive part of our practice and continues to do so. The transformations in our clients' smiles have transformed their lives and it makes me grateful to be part of that process, so much so that we often do veneer cases for free as charitable work for vulnerable individuals.

The Rosenthal course amazed me so much that I wanted to bring it to the UK, so, together with publisher FMC, we organised to bring Larry and his team over and he has run his programme here for several years.

I was also involved in introducing in-surgery tooth whitening to the UK and it continues to be a big part of our practice.

Being in the same practice for so many years has been great, as you get to know generations of clients and see your clinical work from 30 years ago. Reassuringly, the clinical work is still there and functioning well!

Over the last thirty years, alongside my clinical work and work with the BDA, I have also been involved with The British Dental Editors and Writers forum (BEDWF) as a Treasurer Secretary. I also became involved with the Alpha Omega Dental Society, which was originally founded in the US but is now renowned around the world; I have been their International president for several years.

My love and passion for dentistry continues, and I still work clinically four days a week and have recently sold the practice to Dentex.

What is success?

After nearly fifty years in dentistry, if I had to start again and pick a career I would choose dentistry again. For me, that is success!

Top tips for success

Love your patients and love your team.

You must earn the patient's trust; don't just expect it.

Honesty and integrity are vital.

A Game of Two Halves

Julian English
BA (Hons)

Julian English qualified from Leicester University in 1990. Soon after qualifying he joined the newly formed FMC dental publishing company. FMC has now become the leader in dental publishing, events and awards. Julian soon became editorial director at FMC and, with over 23 years of experience working on the award-winning *Dentistry* magazine and numerous other dental journals, he has become a well-known face in the dental world.

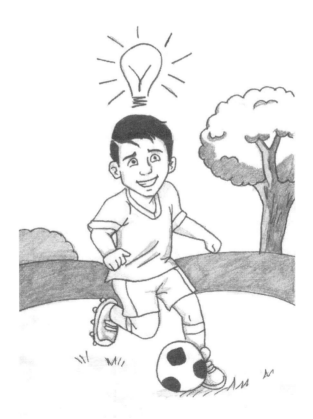

My childhood years were spent in Yorkshire and growing up in a community where there were not many ethnic minorities made life hard. My parents always encouraged me to study hard and to aim for university, as the alternative option would be a life spent down in the coal mines. This was enough motivation for me to excel at school, despite being bullied due to my ethnicity.

I realised early on in my childhood that to make good money meant going to London and this became my goal. I decided to study economics at Leicester University with the eventual aim of becoming a rich stockbroker in London!

As soon as I finished university in 1990, I headed to the bright lights of London; I had no job, no money or a plan but knew this is was where I needed to be. I applied for as many jobs as I could in accountancy and stock brokering but during this time there was a recession, making it impossible to get a job. Companies were downsizing rather than hiring.

I finally managed to get onto a graduate training scheme working in an electrical retail chain shop, which was a tough experience; however, one thing it taught me was how to sell. I also made some good friends at this job and used to play football regularly with these friends on weekends. One of the guys we used to play with also worked on a dental magazine. One day he said he was setting up his own magazine and asked if I would join him in this new venture. At this point I was working for Vodafone in their marketing department writing press releases. It was a fairly dead-end job so I decided to take him up on the offer.

The company was set up in 1995. Since it was a new company and they had no money the job offer was based on me working for no salary for one year! This was too unrealistic for me but eventually I negotiated to work for free for six months rather than a year. Luckily the company took off and within three months I was making money. We only had three of us to begin with and my role started off as an assistant editor. Within 12 months I became editorial director and have stayed on ever since.

What is success?

Success for me is not about money or cars; it's about doing something you like doing that provides you with the lifestyle you want.

Top tips for success

Make friends, keep friends and keep your enemies to a minimum!

From Mouse to Master

Sally Elisabeth Goss
RDS FETC DDHE

Sally Goss is a renowned dental hygienist who has been an inspiration to many within her field. She was the first female and the first hygienist to become president of the British Dental Health Foundation (now called the Oral Health Foundation) and held the position for three years.

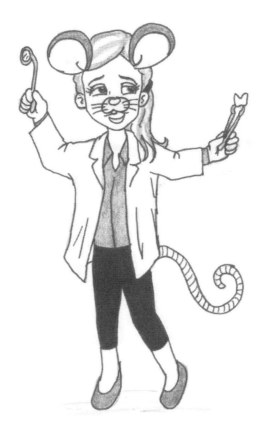

Having left teacher training college and then failing to find a profession which stimulated and excited me, I went to live in Cape Town, South Africa for three years. I went out there as shy and timid as a mouse and returned more confident and more self-assured but still with no idea of my place in the world. And despite there being no history of anyone in the family working in dentistry my mother persuaded me to apply to Dental Hygiene School. In those days you defied your mother at your peril.

In 1975 it was much easier to get into Dental Hygiene School and I was accepted on my first try.   And I discovered to my immense pleasure that this was a job I was born to do. I had finally found a job that was fulfilling and satisfying.

Once I completed my training at St George's Hospital in Tooting I was accepted into the dental department at Marks and Spencer's head office in Baker Street, London. There I was on the top floor of a building that had 3,500 people along with doctors, nurses, hairdressers, chiropodists and other dental staff. It was a great time, and I stayed there for 15 years! The chief dental officer was very supportive of hygienists and I actually ended up marrying him! (Perhaps that was why he was supportive – who knows!) Whilst I was with M&S I presented a paper at the IFDH in Ottawa and I earned my Further Education Teaching Certificate and The Diploma in Dental Health Education. I helped to set up and then administered the M&S Dental Insurance scheme. And I ran a team of 25 hygienists who went into M&S stores on a regular basis to give dental health education to the staff. I also had the privilege of writing a clinical paper with Dr Ruth Freeman. There was, and probably still is, an immense amount of pressure on those staff who choose the merchandise for the various departments of Marks and Spencer and on those who are at the very top end of management. This enabled Ruth and me to publish a joint paper, *'Stress measures as predictors of Periodontal Disease'*, which was published in the Journal of Community Dentistry and Oral Epidemiology.

Whilst at M&S I became aware, through my husband, of the British Dental Health Foundation. I felt a close connection with many of their aims and as I became more involved, my interest grew.

In 1991, M&S offered voluntary redundancy to the majority of employees in Head Office. The offer was too good to refuse and I found myself out of a job with nothing else on the horizon. But luck was on my side. I went to a BSP meeting and happened to sit next to a dentist named Colin Hall Dexter. Colin was very well-known in dentistry; a superb speaker who had revolutionary ideas about patients seeing the hygienist first and getting their oral hygiene perfect before embarking on any other treatments. Bizarrely, his long-term hygienist was about to leave his practice and he was looking for someone to replace her. By the time the BSP meeting was over I had the job of my dreams!

My knowledge and expertise really expanded through working with Colin. Through his recommendation I became the first hygienist to give a presentation in the main hall at a BDA conference. He and I did a roadshow, travelling around giving advice on the most effective ways for hygienist and dentist to work together. It was wonderful to work with someone who valued the hygienist's role. I remember clearly on my first day in his practice he came into my room whilst I was treating a patient and asked me my opinion on the patient's periodontal condition. I looked over my shoulder to see who he was talking to because no dentist had ever asked my opinion before. I had always been told what treatment to carry out. I worked with Colin until he retired.

In 1992, the dentist who was to become my husband and I set up our own practice in Harrow. We worked really well together, and we built a fantastic team. But we were both so involved with other aspects of dentistry that we couldn't commit to the practice full time. Those who own practices know the demands! So we sold the practice.

I was becoming more and more involved in The British Dental Health Foundation (BDHF – now The Oral Health Foundation). I had an idea that the public would benefit from having a helpline that they could phone with any queries on any aspect of dentistry. I set the phone line up in the office in my house, using dental hygienists to provide free and impartial advice on all aspects of dentistry. It quickly became a huge success until eventually it was moved into the BDHF Head Office in Rugby. Since then the helpline has gone from strength to strength and has answered more than 350,000 enquiries. In 1997, I became President of BDHF and stayed in the role for three years. And in 2000 I was given The Probe 'Hygienist of the Year' Award.

I had for a long time been involved with Boots the Chemist. I ran full day seminars teaching staff about products such as toothbrushes, mouthwashes, toothpastes etc. so they could give good advice to the general public. When Boots decided to launch Boots Dental Care in 2000 they invited me to become Hygienist Mentor for all 36 practices – being involved in the recruitment and training of the hygienists. Boots Dental Care were completely supportive of the role of the hygienist within the dental team and understood the importance of patients achieving good gingival health before they embark on extensive dental treatment. Sadly, after five years, just as many of the practices were about to become profitable, Boots decided to close them all down.

Throughout all this time my husband and I had a slot on the radio with BBC Essex in Chelmsford. A friendly chat show was broadcast every afternoon involving knowledgeable people from quite literally all aspects of life. Every six weeks Graham and I would go along and answer phone calls from local people about their dental concerns. It could be quite hair-raising at times because the calls were live so we both had to think on our feet. But it was enormous fun and we continued with the show for almost 20 years.

Throughout my career it was always really important to me that I widened my expertise outside the dental surgery. To that end, I was on the editorial boards of many hygienist journals. I gave multiple presentations – some to small groups such as BDHA and others to much larger groups such as the World Aesthetic Congress at Queen Elizabeth Hall in London. I presented hands-on seminars with a leading periodontist. I have had many articles published in many of the dental journals. Looking back, it has become clear to me how much I have immersed myself in dentistry – it's something I have loved doing. Perhaps being married to a dentist helped!

My husband and I now run our own company, Practice Doctor Ltd. Practice Doctor is a unique practice support package specifically developed to help dentists and their teams cope with the ever more complex operating environment within a dental practice.

What is success?

Knowing your values and sticking to them. Knowing you've done your best with every opportunity that has come your way. Being the best you can possibly be and never settling for 'average'.

Top tips for success

I think luck plays a big part in our lives. Being in the right place at the right time has brought me success in my working life. Nevertheless, pure luck does not sustain you. You have to work hard to maintain your position. Stay current with all aspects of your profession. For instance, when I was working in practice I felt my knowledge of instruments was inadequate, so I booked myself onto a week-long course in San Francisco in the USA. I also contacted a periodontist I knew and worked closely with her for a few weeks to ensure my skills were up to scratch.

Work hard, be patient, spend time with people you admire in the profession and be a sponge for all that learning. Live it ... but above all, love it.

Taste of London

Dr Mark Hughes
BA BDentSC (Dubl)

Dr Mark Hughes qualified from Dublin's Trinity College in 1992. Mark is a strong advocate for patient-centred dentistry and over the years he has designed, developed and managed many high end private cosmetic dental practices including the Harley Street Dental Group. Mark enjoys both the clinical and business sides of dentistry. He is now a partner in Dentex, which is a business that involves co-ownership of multiple practices with the aim of improving the running of practices and growing them.

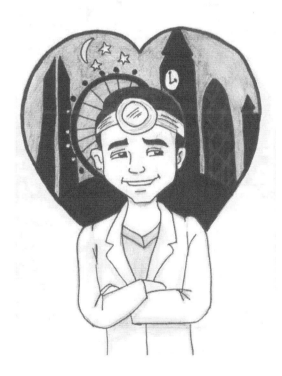

During my time at secondary school in Dublin there was a big emphasis on eventually becoming a professional. The nature of education pushed us towards getting a stable professional career, especially given the economic climate in Ireland at that time. I decided on a career in dentistry and after school I got a place at Trinity College to study dentistry.

After qualifying in 1992 there were not many opportunities in Ireland, so, like a lot of Irish people of my generation, I came to the UK. Initially my plan was to stay in the UK for a few months, get some experience and then move back home; this plan never materialised!

I got my first job at an NHS practice in Essex and I realised very quickly it was not for me. I wanted to be in London and experience London life, plus a lot of my friends from Ireland had moved to London. Six months later I managed to move to central London and got a job in South London. Through a university connection I was lucky to get a flat share in the heart of Chelsea and really experience London life. I got a taste of London life at the very high end and there was no going back!

The practice I worked in was a busy NHS practice located in Streatham. I gained lots of experience working there and at the same time had a great time, as the principal and associate were fun and were well connected with clubs, bars and restaurants. I was living a life that I had never dreamt of and even managed to get on the property ladder with a flat in Battersea.

At the age of twenty-six I began to yearn for travel. I wanted a break from all the years of studying followed by going straight into work. I decided to rent my flat and travelled around the world for nearly two years, including visiting South America, the USA, Australia, Indonesia, Thailand, Cambodia, Vietnam and New Zealand. In Australia I managed to get a job with the Flying Doctors, which was an amazing experience. A slightly more terrifying experience was being caught up in the middle of a military coup in Jakarta; luckily, we were evacuated out quickly! After 18 months of travelling I decided I was ready to come back to London and get back into my career.

Once I got back from travelling I knew I wanted to buy a dental practice and eventually purchased a practice in Covent Garden, after working in it as an associate for a while. Immediately I invested heavily into the practice and refurbished it to a high standard. I also invested in website marketing, which, at that time, was a relatively new concept in the dental world.

During this time, I was also attending lots of dental courses in the UK and USA, including Larry Rosenthal in New York, The Pankey Institute in Miami and Invisalign. I enjoyed cosmetic dentistry and wanted to focus on a career in this area.

In 2003 another opportunity came to purchase a dental practice at 42 Harley Street from a retiring principal; it was a one surgery practice with a flat above, allowing me to live rent free, with the prospect of expanding the practice into the flat once it got busier. I embarked on another refurbishment project, this time taking it to another level and designing the practice to give it the 'Wow' factor. My focus was to make this look like no other dental practice. Seeing so much potential here made me decide to sell my practice in Covent Garden and focus on Harley Street.

This focus allowed me to grow the business from a one-surgery to a three-surgery practice. Fourteen years on we now have a whole building, 4500 square feet, and have grown to nine dental surgeries with over thirty people working there. During this time there were highs and lows – including the financial crash in 2008 – but we managed to get through the difficult times.

It was in 2008 that I met my business partner with the vision to develop and grow the main practice and also purchase other practices. This partnership led to purchasing multiple practices over the next few years, leading to the creation of the Harley Street Dental Group. Our practices included one in the City of London, Chelsea and another one in Harley Street. Before long we also realised we had outgrown our main practice at 42 Harley Street and needed to find a bigger building. Fortunately, we were offered 52 Harley Street by Harold de Walden, who owns the majority of freeholds on Harley Street. We embarked on another massive refurbishment project, this time helped by the landlord, who invested almost £1.5 million into the building; this whole process took two years in the planning and execution.

Moving five doors down seemed simple enough but was the biggest headache of my life! We had to complete the whole move over one weekend to ensure we could open the practice on Monday morning in the new location. The first few years were difficult as the extra expenses had a big impact on the business; however, since then the practice has continued to become more and more successful.

I soon discovered that trying to grow a group of practices was not only challenging dealing with the number of people involved, but also with basic infrastructure it becomes very difficult. To make it a success you need a marketing team, financial team, bookkeeping team, training team, procurement and acquisitions team. We also had difficulty getting lending from the banks to purchase further practices as it was only the two partners, and the banks could not understand how we could manage any further practices. To get to the corporate level in terms of lending was impossible so I looked at other ways of doing this including venture capital, private investments, fund managers and eventually this gave rise to the creation of Dentex.

What is success?

Making a positive difference in people's lives, not only patients but also your colleagues.

Top tips for success

Communication is key, not just in dentistry but in life!

Have a clear set of goals. Think of what you are trying to achieve and why you are trying to achieve it and follow your dreams.

Always remember our profession is here to serve and help people. If you stick to this principle the success will come.

Be Interested in Everything

Dr Ian Hutchinson
BDS, FDS, RCSED, MOrth, Msc

Dr Ian Hutchinson qualified from Newcastle University in 1991 and worked his way through various hospital posts covering all disciplines of dentistry as well as working in NHS general practice. Following this, he embarked on his Orthodontic Specialist training in Bristol between 1996-1999. Ian was chairman of the British Lingual Orthodontic Society (2015-2017) and serves on the editorial board of the *European Journal of Orthodontics*. He founded Warwick University's MSc in Lingual Orthodontics and runs his own orthodontic courses in Labial and Lingual Orthodontics. Ian is a big advocate for interdisciplinary dentistry and has a passion for the synergy that exists between orthodontics and restorative dentistry.

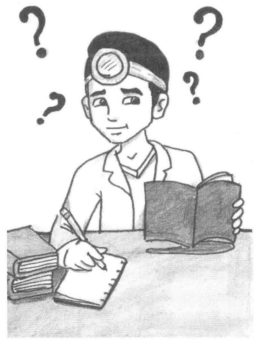

I always liked 'fiddling', or working with my hands, and fell into a dental degree in 1986 at Newcastle University. For me it was a challenging degree, as I would say I'm not the brightest bulb in the box and reading and writing is not my strong point. Over the years I've come to learn that I am a 'visual' person and combined with being a 'plodder' I muddled through. To break the 'death by PowerPoint' I'd dream about riding my bike and often escape into the physiology department to be their 'lab rat'. After qualifying, I stayed on in Newcastle for a house officer job in prosthetics, which was followed by an SHO maxillofacial and orthodontic post in Coventry and Warwick Hospital; a baptism of fire 'one in two'... (If you truly want to learn then 'total immersion' is the way to go and being on call every other night in a busy trauma unit you learn a lot ... and quick!)

During my time as an SHO I found the orthodontists were friendly and approachable whereas the maxillofacial consultants were quite the opposite. Fortunately my sharp reflexes helped me avoid flying instruments and the wrapping of the knuckles! I learnt to 'suck it up', as they say. The flip side (there's always a flip side to everything) was that I gained a lot of experience and how to 'think on your feet'. Another essential lesson that has remained is the importance of patient communication. Communication is a two-way process. Unfortunately we don't listen to patients enough; we are all too keen to jump in and 'do something' when instead, taking time to listen and allowing the story to unfold, the patient will tell you what's wrong with them. Dentistry is not just learning to 'read the teeth', it's about listening as well.

At this stage I was still undecided whether to specialise in orthodontics or maxillofacial surgery and decided more experience of other aspects of dentistry would be useful. I was fortunate to gain a rotational SHO job around Birmingham which covered more max fax (but with much more oncology), restorative, oral medicine and orthodontics. I also worked at Birmingham Children's Hospital, which was both an amazing and humbling experience. During this time, I started in NHS general dental practice, working evenings and Saturdays.

After three years of the rotation, I decided I did not want to do another five years of university (to read medicine) so decided to specialise in orthodontics. Getting a specialist training post proved very difficult. At this point I had moved into full time NHS general practice and after just over a year of applying for *any* ortho training position, on my 11th attempt I got a place on the Bristol training programme. I think they regretted it as I could never stop myself asking: "But why?", which irritated the life out of one professor in particular … but if you can't explain by painting a mental picture then don't teach! I continued to pour fuel on the fire by working evenings in the emergency dental clinic (as I love taking teeth out…) while the 'ivory tower' expected us to be home every night studying and writing essays. Did I mention I'm a stubborn bugger…?

Following my specialist training I got a locum consultant job in Solihull, which I enjoyed. I even participated in ward rounds with the oral surgeons, as despite being an orthodontist I was still interested in getting my fingers wet doing other things apart from bending wire. It's important to appreciate how all the disciplines interact closely with each other, and by doing so you learn more.

After the consultant job I worked in a specialist orthodontic practice on the NHS, whilst at the same time doing the odd maxillofacial locum job as I still enjoyed it.

I then strayed into the 'practice ownership' den. I purchased an orthodontic practice with a couple of colleagues. I made the fatal mistake of assuming that we all shared similar values. Unfortunately, how can I put it… Someone stole all the cookies from the jar. This was stressful to say the least and led to four years of legal battles with barristers where I learnt a lesson: trust is one of the most important things and you must have your values aligned. With hindsight, maybe I should have rolled over. Life is too short, especially when you measure time differently (think about how many summers you have left…) but once I get my teeth into something I don't let go. Know what makes you tick, what type of person are you and learn to manage it – or I should say learn to manage yourself and your chimp.

From this experience I decided to set up a private squat practice in Chepstow, on my own. After the legal battle I also ended up with the NHS orthodontic practice and so began the process of running between the two practices, managing them both, plus doing all my lab work on a Sunday! This is the point when I realised the importance of working on the business, and not in the business. It is impossible to work five days clinically and then on top of that run your own business; it becomes a recipe for major stress and eventually leads to disaster.

At a business coaching group I bumped into a lab technician, Sue Beasant. We decided to set up an orthodontic laboratory together called Wired Orthodontics. At this point my teaching career also started. I had a few friends who wanted to learn orthodontics so I taught them and then they referred their friends, who then referred their friends and from there it snowballed.

I recently passed over the NHS practice to focus more on the private practice and teaching. I have always been a keen advocate for interdisciplinary dentistry, as this is the only way to achieve the best long term and aesthetic result for the patient, and this has led me to continue my education into other disciplines in dentistry. I love listening to Frank Spear: he has experience, he has stories to tell, and he sees the synergy between ortho and restorative dentistry.

What is success?

Success to me is freedom ... freedom from financial pressures and time constraints. Freedom to think, grow and be happy and make others happy. Freedom to pass on everything I've learnt to the next generation.

Success is not about big shiny objects.

Top tips for success

Be interested in everything and experience everything.

Dentistry can be a very rewarding career but also at times very stressful. Ensure you look after yourself and your wellbeing, and I don't just mean physically either. In the words of Laird Hamilton, "make sure your worst enemy doesn't live between your own two ears."

Time management is critical for success; you must balance your time of working in the business and on the business.

Never, ever stop learning and keep an open mind as theories and treatments can change over time, especially with the advent of new technology allowing us to view things from a different perspective.

Don't get distracted or be made to feel inferior by the antics of some on social media. Keep your head down, get your work done, get the experience and be the best you can.

In the words of Henry Ford, "if you think you can or if you think you can't, you are right."

Sliding Doors

Dr Zaki Kanaan

BDS, MSc, DipDSed, LFHom

Dr Zaki Kanaan qualified from Guy's Hospital in 1996. He found his main passion in implant dentistry and obtained his master's degree in 2001 from Guy's Hospital. Zaki also has a big interest in cosmetic dentistry and has been a past president of the British Academy of Cosmetic Dentistry (BACD). He also has a Diploma in Sedation, a Diploma in Hypnosis and is a Licentiate of the Faculty of Homeopathy. Zaki has received numerous awards, the highlight of which was being voted UK Dentist of the Year at the Dental Awards in 2012 and being given the Outstanding Contribution to Private Dentistry Award in 2014. As well as spending his time on the lecture circuit, Zaki owns an implant and aesthetic private practice with his wife in Fulham and is on the board of the Association of Dental Implantology (ADI).

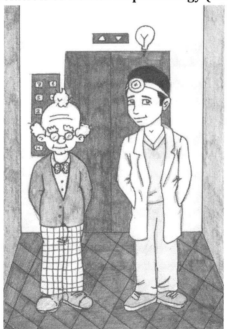

Born in Beirut, my family made the decision to move to the UK when I was three years old. After schooling I decided on becoming a dentist.

University was a great time for me; it was here where I would, without knowing it, meet my future wife, Dominique. After qualifying from Guy's Hospital in 1996 I completed my vocational training and headed out in search of a private job. I went to over 20 interviews and got a rejection each time based on my lack of experience, youth and lack of having anything special to offer. After this experience I decided I needed to get some further qualifications and quickly. The quickest option was a Diploma in Sedation at Guy's Hospital. Once I obtained the Diploma in 1998, I went back to searching for private jobs with a more positive outlook and due to my new-found skill of providing sedation I landed many offers. I had found a niche in the dental world, which was my way in to a career in private dentistry.

Although my Diploma in Sedation taught me a lot, it never went into the detail of talking and communicating with patients so I started looking into hypnosis and found it very interesting, ultimately deciding to do a Diploma in Hypnosis with my wife. During this course I experienced for myself the feeling of no pain whilst being injected under hypnosis. That was when I became a true believer in mind over matter!

Having realised the importance of extra qualifications I began thinking of doing a restorative master's degree; however, this all changed when I had a casual meeting in a lift. Whilst studying at Guy's Hospital for the sedation diploma I bumped into Professor Richard Palmer, who was running the Implant MSc at Guy's. Professor Palmer convinced me to apply for the implant rather than the restorative course. This inopportune meeting in the lift paved the way to my career in implant dentistry. Professor Palmer's words made sense; he told me: "You can already do restorative work. The master's degree will make you better at restorative, but why not offer something you don't already do, such as implants?"

After having a long hard think about what Professor Palmer had said to me, I decided to apply for the implant master's degree, managed to get a place in 1999 and completed the degree in 2001. Looking back, this was the best thing I ever did.

An Implant Msc in 2001 was quite rare back then and this opened up many new job offers in a variety of different private practices in

London, including James Goolnik's Bow Lane practice in the city, where I was predominantly going in to provide implant treatment. Another practice that my wife and I worked in was Ora Dental in Selfridges.

After the success of the first BACD conference I applied to be elected onto the board and I managed to get on (after a few attempts!). After eight years on the board doing various roles, I became the president of the BACD in 2013. Soon after leaving the BACD I was approached to be a board member of the ADI, which was actually a better fit because of my passion for implant dentistry.

In 2008 my wife and I decided to take the plunge and set up our own small private practice from scratch in Fulham: K2 Dental. During this time, it also became legal for hygienists and therapists to carry out whitening treatments; our hygienists wanted to do these treatments but found no available courses. We decided to run an in-house course at the practice for our hygienists and following the success of this course we received requests to run further whitening courses, both for hygienists at our practice and other practices. Eventually I was approached by Philips when they took over Discuss Dental to help with the tooth whitening part of their business.

I currently work part time at our practice and two others, as well as lecturing and running a year-long implant course with two colleagues, working with Philips and being part of the ADI. All of this has only been achievable with the help of my wife. Even though we qualified together, Dominique has allowed me to continue with my career and obtain further qualifications whilst she focused more on the family and running and managing our practice, and for that I am forever grateful.

What is success?

Doing what you love to do and being well respected and well known amongst your peers and your patients.

Top tips for success

Find your niche in the dental world. This gives you your unique selling point; companies need a unique selling point but so do individuals. If you do exactly what everyone else does you won't stand out from the crowd.

Never say no, always say yes and think about the offer after. By saying no straight away you limit your choices immediately. Life is like sliding doors: you always get a choice but the key is having the time to think it over and make the right choice. These choices will shape your life, just like my experience with Professor Palmer in the lift.

Best of Both Worlds

Dr Tony Kilcoyne
BDS, LDS, MGDSRCS (Eng), M.Med.Sci (U.Sheff), FFGDP (UK)

Dr Tony Kilcoyne graduated from the University of Sheffield in 1983. Since qualifying, Tony has followed a dual career pathway both in the general dental and hospital setting. Tony is a specialist prosthodontist with a specialist practice in Yorkshire. For over 27 years he has been the dental foundation training programme director for the Dewsbury scheme. Previously, Tony was a clinical teacher, clinical supervisor and lecturer. He has also been on the board of the General Dental Council (GDC) and is currently on the board of the British Dental Association (BDA).

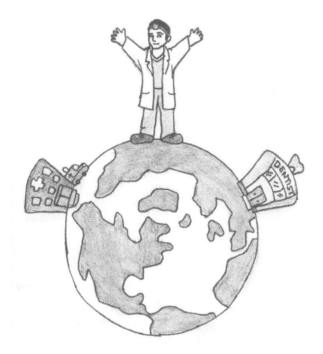

At the age of eighteen I had two career choices in mind; these were to become an actuary leading to work in the insurance industry, or to work in the health profession. I eventually decided on applying for medicine. Following my application, the more I researched into a career in medical practice the more I began thinking it was not the right choice for me. At this point I started looking into a career in dentistry and found that it ticked more practical boxes for me than medicine. Unfortunately, by now my university applications had already been sent in for medicine.

I decided to take the initiative and call all the dental schools directly, explaining how I no longer wanted to do medicine and that dentistry was the right career choice for me. Luckily a few of those schools did invite me in for an interview. Sheffield University offered me a provisional place, if a place became available. Just days before the start of the course I received a letter from them advising a place had become available and that I had been accepted! This was brilliant news and I accepted the offer, but it made for a manic rushed start to my dental career!

My time at Sheffield was amazing. The dental school was very good, the teaching at the university was perfect for a GDP and in 1983 I qualified with my BDS. At that time vocational training was only just beginning so most of the graduates, including me, went out searching for a supporting practice that helped mentor the young graduate. I decided to come back to my home town of Bradford and found a lovely supporting practice where I worked for a while, followed by another associate job in Bradford.

At this point I was also looking for somewhere to live and stumbled on a beautiful village named Haworth about eight miles outside Bradford. Driving around this lovely place I started looking at properties and randomly stumbled on a hairdresser's for sale. As soon as I saw this property I thought it would be an ideal place for a dental practice. After doing some research into the area, I was advised by the NHS they had been wanting a dentist in this village for some time. Even though I had only been qualified for a few years I decided to take the plunge and applied for planning permission to convert the hairdresser's into a dental practice. This proved more difficult than I thought as other dentists soon started competing with me for the site once planning went public. I decided to contact the seller directly and managed to strike a deal with them, as long as we completed the deal in six weeks! The pressure was on and we struggled on to the last minute but managed to complete in time. I now had to embark on a major renovation project to convert the site into a functioning dental practice. To make life even harder, in those days we could not even advertise so I had to advertise by word of mouth in and around the village. Once the practice was open, I worked there part time whilst still carrying on with my associate job until the practice slowly became busier. At this point the practice was one hundred percent NHS.

During this time, I saw a part time job advertised for a clinical supervisor at the local dental school. Since the practice was still slightly quiet I decided to apply for this position and went in for the interview with low expectations as I had only been qualified for three years. To my surprise I was offered the job on the spot, right after my interview.

On my first day I was very nervous and shadowed a consultant who wanted to show me the ropes. His style of teaching was shockingly authoritarian to say the least, and this immediately relieved my anxiety as I realised that, even though I was not that experienced, my teaching ability would be constructive! I soon began to love being a supervisor, getting great satisfaction from teaching and helping the students as much as possible through the stresses and challenges ahead.

As my career progressed I began to do more postgraduate qualifications plus some part time specialist prosthodontic training courses in hospital. Seventeen years of this part time experience eventually got me onto the General Dental Council's specialist prosthodontic list. I enjoyed the mix of working in general practice and at the hospital, getting the best of both worlds. I believe my patients have had better care from me, my teaching ability has improved, my skills have improved, I have obtained further qualifications, all as a result of being involved in both the general dental practice setting and hospital setting.

As my skill set grew I realised I could not provide all this specialist treatment and spend the time I wanted to with my patients on the NHS, so in 1991 when the contract was changing for the worst (cuts), my practice went to predominantly private and we kept seeing children on the NHS. The NHS element gradually disappeared and by about 1998 the practice was fully private and specialised in prosthodontics.

Along the way came another teaching opportunity to become a foundation trainer, which I did for several years in practice. Then, in 1991, I applied to be the training programme director to run the vocational training scheme, which meant giving up my undergraduate teaching role. I have now been a VT Advisor/DFTPD for over twenty-seven years!

Between 2003 and 2009 I also became elected to the General Dental Council by the profession and then when systems changed to centralised appointments, was appointed to the GDC board again between 2009 and 2013. I enjoyed this experience as it meant I could give the GDC some real-world perspective to the professional regulations. Unfortunately, in 2013 I had to leave as the GDC had a rule of not being able to do more than two terms in a ten-year period. It was very sad to see it go downhill after that.

One of my passions is oral health education and I am an active campaigner for prevention and improved child dental health in the national media.

In January 2017 I was voted onto the BDA PEC board, which is an overall strategic board that controls the BDA. With the BDA I am trying to improve the current situation and systems for the profession, particularly for newly qualified dentists, the future leaders of our profession.

What is success?

You are truly successful when you learn to know yourself; you can control your own destiny and continually improve in many ways.

Top tips for success

Know your strengths and your weaknesses and focus on improving upon your weaknesses, to at least neutralise, then develop them.

Remember almost everything started as a weakness!

Try to find an environment to work in where you are happy and be a part of perpetuating that happy environment too.

Have a good work and life balance; we work to live, we don't live to work.

Create time to talk to patients and communicate with them to provide patient-centred care.

Be kind to yourself as well as others; be the change you'd like to see, realistically.

New York, New York

Ashley Latter

Ashley Latter has become a household name within the dental profession. He has delivered over 23,000 hours of business coaching to the dental industry all over the world, including his most famous Ethical Sales and Communication course. In 2014 Ashley was voted number 12 in the top 150 most influential people in UK dentistry.

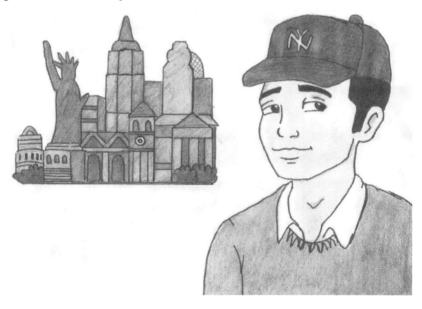

My story starts twenty-six years ago when I started working with the Dale Carnegie Training Organisation. A year before this, I took the Dale Carnegie course, which I loved. I took the course as my confidence was low and I didn't like the job I was in. The course was truly inspirational and increased my confidence and communication skills. At that point I had a well-paid job in banking but I hated it. I decided to leave the world of banking and plunge into a new career working within the Dale Carnegie Organisation, selling and delivering their course programmes in Manchester on a commission only basis.

The first year selling programmes was very tough. My income

dropped massively from my days in banking; I was barely making enough to survive and was relying on credit cards. After the first year I was contemplating giving up selling the courses and going back into finance. However, one day in my office I received a fax advertising a course in New York run by the number one top seller of courses out of fifteen hundred members in the entire Dale Carnegie organisation.

I decided to stick some more money on my credit card and flew to New York to attend the three-day course. This course was incredible; it changed the way I thought about selling. Rather than just trying to sell the courses, I needed to find out what the clients' true wants and needs were. This course changed my life!

When I got back from the course I put what I had learned into practice. Within a year I had quadrupled my sales and another year later I became the number one salesperson in the UK and stayed number one for the next eight years. I became top five in the world and an international master trainer, going around the world training trainers to become trainers.

In 1997 two dentists, along with other sales people from various industries, took one of my sales courses. I couldn't figure out why two dentists were there and as they left I told them I would call them for a follow up.

A few weeks later I was lying on my couch wondering how those dentists had got on after the course. I was debating whether I should call them or not but eventually decided to and I'm glad I did! I discovered that prior to the course they were struggling communicating and selling treatments to patients but following my course their treatment plan uptakes had increased. For the first time ever they were delivering the type of dentistry they loved and, more importantly, what the patients wanted.

Those two dentists told their friends about the course, which led to my first ever Ethical Sales and Communication course twenty-two years ago in Oxford, in front of twenty-six dentists. After the course I did follow up calls with all the dentists and they all said the same thing: their treatment plan acceptance had increased, more patients were saying yes and they were doing more of the dentistry they loved.

From those two dentists to now has been an incredible journey. We have had over seventeen thousand dentists worldwide take the Ethical Sales and Communication course in fourteen different countries. I have also been involved in writing four books and various online courses. We now also deliver courses to other dental team members including practice managers, receptionists and entrepreneurs.

What is success?

Doing what you love every day, from waking up in the morning with the person you love, to going to work and getting paid well for doing something you love.

Top tips for success

Be a people person and build relationships with people.

Have excellent communication and listening skills.

Learning how to sell without selling.

Be positive and persistent.

Always be pushing yourself. Never take anything for granted. Never stop doing the things that made you successful in the first place.

Never stop learning: the more you learn, the more you earn!

A True East-ender!

Mr David McAnerney
BDS (Hons), BSc (Hons), MBBS, MFDS, FRCS, PGCE (Med ed)

David McAnerney qualified in 2005 from The Royal London. David had a real passion for oral surgery and whilst at university decided to specialise in Oral and Maxillo-Facial Surgery (OMFS). After further qualifying in medicine, he went on to become a registrar in the East of England and is aiming to obtain his consultancy in 2018.

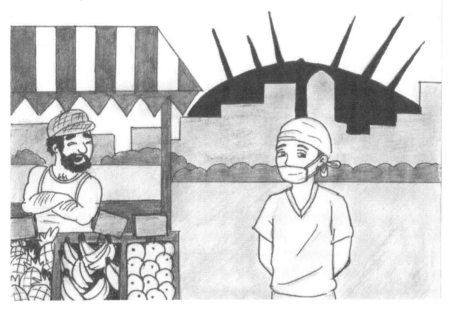

Growing up, I was surrounded by the medical and dental world: my grandfather was a doctor, my father was a dentist and my mother had been an ITU nurse. After completing some work experience at my father's practice, my aim was to follow in my father's footsteps and become a dentist. Even now I consider myself as a dentist rather than a doctor or surgeon.

After applying for dentistry, I choose to go to the Royal London and studied dentistry in 1999. Between my fourth and fifth year I decided to do an intercalated BSc as I wanted a break from dentistry and also wanted to learn and see something different. I chose to do oral biology and really enjoyed it, particularly research.

During my time at university, I began to look into sub-specialising and I always had a great love for oral surgery. Rather than doing sports on a Wednesday afternoon I would join the max-fax team and observe them in clinics and in theatre, during which time my interest grew further. That's not to say I was averse to sports, as I was the president of the QMUL Chinese kickboxing society and an avid indoor rock climber.

After qualifying in 2005, I decided to do vocational training to keep my options open instead of going straight back to hospital. Working in general practice was a great experience. I loved the dentistry as well as the patient interaction, but I always felt I wanted to do more, so I decided to go back to hospital and take on an SHO (Senior House Officer) post at the Royal London. It was during this time I finally decided I wanted to do OMFS so I applied for medicine.

I managed to get onto the three-year accelerated medical course back at the Royal London. I was becoming a true East-ender! At that time, I had a family so to fund myself through the degree and help financially, I was a clinical fellow for Whipps Cross and Harlow during the three years, which meant a lot of on calls and late nights, on top of studying for the medical degree. However, this is very much the standard for anyone wishing to pursue this course of training.

After qualifying in medicine I then had to go through the process of the foundation years and core surgical training, which I completed in the East of England training scheme. During this time, I chose specialities that were related to, or work alongside OMFS, such as anaesthetics, ENT and plastics.

Following on from this, I applied for a registrar position in OMFS in the East of England and got it. Over many years, I have completed all the rotations, travelling from one hospital to another and completing all areas of training. Now I am finally ready to become a consultant! My journey began in 1999, and after many years of hard work has led to my consultancy in 2018. It has been a long, hard but enjoyable journey with some sacrifices along the way, particularly with regards to spending time with my family. Becoming a consultant now allows me to finally settle down in one location, with my family around me.

What is success?

When I was at the beginning of my training, I would have defined success through academic and surgical achievements. However, now, coming towards the end of my training, my success would be a happy work/life balance. To be fulfilled at work is important but to be fulfilled at home is equally important.

Top tips for success

Always set a goal, have a plan and go for it!

The Envelope Plan

Dr Christopher Orr
BSc, BDS

Dr Christopher Orr graduated from Queen's University, Belfast, in 1996 and he is one of the UK's most prominent aesthetic and cosmetic dentists. He is a past president and accredited member of the British Academy of Cosmetic Dentistry, a former director of the American Academy of Cosmetic Dentistry, a certified member of the European Society of Cosmetic Dentistry and a certified member of the British Dental Bleaching Society. Since 2008, he is also the head of judges for the Aesthetic Dentistry Awards, which promotes outstanding dentistry done for patients throughout UK.

As course director of Advanced Dental Seminars (ADS), he has run the UK's most established one-year programme on cosmetic dentistry and aesthetic restorative dentistry for dentists from all over the UK and Europe. He divides his working time between training dentists and treating patients at his state-of-the-art practice and training facility in London Bridge. He also regularly travels abroad to attend and lecture at professional conferences.

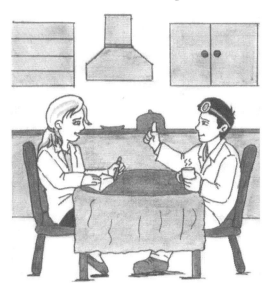

At university I was involved with international dental student organisations and became the president for both the International Dental Students' Association (IADS) and European Dental Students (EDS). It was a lot of fun being involved with these organisations and it allowed me to travel the world and meet lots of interesting people – including my wife, Zeynep. On my travels to various dental schools and dental practices around the world, I learnt dentistry is very similar wherever you go, but what is different is how you do it.

At a meeting in Hong Kong, I met Sverker Toreskog, who at the time was one of the most innovative dentists in the world. Seeing what he was doing made me realise that there was a lot more to dentistry than what we were being taught at university.

After qualifying in 1996, I moved to England. The plan was to do my VT training, then learn more about restorative dentistry and go back to Belfast. My VT year was in Maidstone and my trainer was brilliant. He taught me a lot, but I did find working on the NHS very frustrating.

It was at this time my love affair with the camera started. I began to take a lot of photographs of my work. After VT, I found a job in Old Street at a sedation-based practice, dealing with anxious patients. At this practice I began to look at and treat the patient's whole mouth, rather than focusing on single tooth dentistry.

Following from there, I was lucky enough to get my first fully private job. I wasn't sure how I got the job but was grateful for the opportunity! On reflection, I definitely think having a portfolio of before and after case photos helped as it was not at all common at the time. Here I began to do some of the more adventurous conservative and adhesive types of dentistry that I had learnt from Sverker. I also learnt how to manage failure and patients' expectations as unfortunately the associate who I had taken over from had left recent work that was already failing. Going through the process of successfully fixing these failures made me more confident of dealing with my future failures.

I was enjoying my time at this practice and loving the type of dentistry I was doing, but then the practice was sold to a corporate and the new owners offered me a 40% pay cut and a salary! I had to move on and applied for a job with a small group of cosmetic dental practices based in London called Dentics. Again, I went to the interview with my big portfolio of photos and managed to convince them to give me a job! This was late 1990s, early 2000s and London was full of young adults who were relapsed ortho cases. Retention was not provided as a long-term treatment and no short-term ortho or clear aligner systems were available at the time. GDPs had not started offering ortho treatments themselves to patients. These patients would not consider further orthodontic treatment as it usually involved two to three years of fixed appliances. As far as they were concerned, ortho had failed. So we used to get a lot of veneer cases and I realised that I needed to learn more.

I began by going to the US regularly, mainly to the American Academy of Cosmetic Dentistry (AACD) meetings. These meetings were always inspirational and taught me so much. Dentics were very supportive of me learning more and allowed me to travel to numerous other courses around the world to learn from the best, including Peter Dawson, Frank Spear, Pascal Magne, Newton Fahl and many more. Working in a cosmetic practice allowed me to put into practice everything I was learning. What I was doing on a day-to-day basis had become very different to the general dentistry of the times and I began to get requests from other dentists who wanted to come and see the way I worked and learn from me. I do not believe you can learn much from watching someone do the work in the surgery unless you understand how and why it is done in the first place. This was the start of me trying to figure out how to share my knowledge with others.

Unfortunately, Dentics was also sold to a bigger corporate! The new company appointed me as their clinical director. The role became very challenging and led to a lot of frustration in dealing with individuals who did not understand dentistry. Not surprisingly, they did not last long and were bought by yet another corporate. It was time for me to leave.

I was fed up with the corporate world of dentistry and decided it was time to set up my own practice. A two-surgery practice came up for sale in Covent Garden with a studio flat above it included in the sale. The plan was to work as two dentists with Zeynep at the practice and run a course once a month, upstairs in the flat.

Early in 2003, one Saturday morning, we were chatting after

breakfast. The idea of setting up our own course to teach others had been on our minds for a while. With the pile of new post sitting by our side, I lifted a big white envelope and we literally planned the whole course on the back of it!

The programme was designed to teach aesthetic and cosmetic restorative dentistry to dentists over the course of a year. We made up a simple brochure and, with the help of our technician friends, sent it out to their customers. We did not know if anyone would trust us, but they did! Bookings started coming along but the practice purchase fell through, leaving us with thirty dentists who wanted to attend the course but no venue to run it from! We were humbled and very grateful by the number of dentists willing to take our first ever course and did not want to disappoint them.

Luckily, we found a seminar room for rent in Harley Street. There was no way we could teach 30 people in a class properly, so we divided them into two groups on our first year. On the second year we had to double up to four groups as our first-year delegates signed up their husbands, wives, associates, friends... It was truly overwhelming.

The idea of setting up the British Academy of Cosmetic Dentistry (BACD) had always been on my mind since going to the AACD meetings. With the help of AACD's UK member list, I arranged a meeting in November 2003 and invited anyone vaguely interested in setting up the BACD to come. In its first year it was run from our living room and I led the academy for four years as president. Now after all these years it is very satisfying to see the growth and influence BACD has had in the UK dental profession.

In terms of teaching at ADS, year on year, the number of dentists wanting to do the course increased and it became more and more popular. We had principals who would sign up all their associates or would only employ people who had done the 'Chris Orr course'. What started off as a fun plan, running a course once a month, had now become a massive commitment, but still was and is fun. Zeynep took full time management of the courses and I continued to work clinically at a few different practices in London.

A couple years of running courses in rented rooms proved to us that we needed a better facility to improve what we were giving to our delegates. Doing practical sessions in hotel rooms, which are not equipped to have suctions, proper lighting, motors was frustrating to us. No private teaching facility of the standards we wanted existed in the UK at the time, so we decided to build our own.

Zeynep convinced me to come south of the river, which took a lot of persuading as I used to remember it as a very rough and run-down area. However, it was undergoing a massive redevelopment programme and we found an old warehouse on Bermondsey Street, which was just a shell. She hired a building firm and focused on designing the warehouse into a postgraduate dental education facility with a dental practice. She managed and supervised this massive project of opening the largest privately-owned dental training facility at the time.

We started the new course sessions in October 2008 in our new facility. The course continues to be popular and we are very proud to be running it continuously without any marketing since the start. ADS Alumni, dentists who have finished the year programme, are a wonderful bunch who are proud to be associated with us. Our relationship with them continues after the sessions finish.

Of course, we make a conscious effort to regularly update the course every year with new material. I believe if you stop learning, you should stop teaching. Everything I learn goes into my teaching.

Dentistry has evolved hugely over the last 15 years with new technology, materials and systems. The boundaries of specialist topics moved into the realm of general practitioners. This is making everyday dentistry more enjoyable but requires more regular and up to date training.

As a teacher my objective is to guide colleagues into the unknown and get rid of the dogma and doubt. Simplify the information overload and make them confident individuals. The number of alumni members popping up in the professional awards or on the lecture circuit shows me that I am doing it right.

I also still work clinically at the practice, taking on more challenging cases that have been referred to us, with a team of in-house specialists to provide the best results. Helping our patients with their dental problems and teaching my colleagues what I do in practice is the best of both worlds for me.

What is success?

Success is contentment. Are you happy with where you are and what you are doing in life?

Top tips for success

Success doesn't happen overnight; it takes time. Be patient and listen. Listen to your mentors, your peers but most importantly, your patients.

And of course, get a camera and use it!

The Reincarnation

Dr Ashish B Parmar
BDS (Lond.)

Dr Ash Parmar qualified in 1991 from Guy's Hospital. Since qualifying, Ash has invested heavily in postgraduate training and has become an internationally respected dentist with a special interest in cosmetic dentistry. Motivated and inspired to deliver the best possible smile makeovers and dental care, Ash works very closely with his patients to embark on the journey together, at his state-of-the-art practice in Chigwell, Essex. It is one of the most technologically advanced practices in the UK. Alongside his passion for clinical dentistry, Ash runs several dental courses and has mentored countless dentists over his career. Ash is humble in his personal life and has a firm commitment to ongoing personal and spiritual development and charitable support, all with a structured work/life balance.

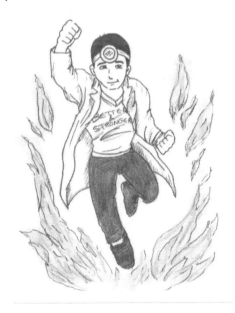

I have always had a passion for dentistry and after qualifying in 1991, I was ready to embark on my new exciting career! I completed my VT training at a practice in Chingford, which was a great experience; I even stayed on as a part time associate for a few years after. At that time, I also began working part time in a predominantly NHS practice in Enfield, which provided me with a good experience.

Following this I decided to go into partnership with Rahul Doshi and to purchase a practice. I met Rahul at university and ever since then we have been good friends. The first practice we purchased was in Hornchurch. It was a mixed practice but was also rundown and had a lot of potential. The first year was tough as being a principal was a steep learning curve on top of gaining the trust of the patients. Following a refurbishment, we slowly learnt the ropes and the practice started doing well. Our wives, who are both dentists, treated the NHS patients, whilst Rahul and I saw the private patients.

As things were going well, we decided to buy another small practice, this time in Barnet. A few years later we decided to purchase practice number three in Hertford (a squat practice). Without knowing, this would eventually become our flagship practice.

A big turning point in my career came in the nineties, when Larry Rosenthal came to the UK and we did a day course with him. It was such an inspirational course and showed us a whole new level of dentistry. Larry was a very passionate speaker; his passion rubbed off on me and from that point I knew I wanted to be a cosmetic dentist. Since I was mainly seeing private patients in our practices, I knew I could deliver cosmetic dentistry. All I needed to do now was to learn it!

The first course we did was a hands-on smile makeover course delivered by Larry Rosenthal at the Eastman Dental Institute. This was a great learning experience: we were thrown in at the deep end and did a smile makeover during the course. This gave us the hunger to do more so we took his level 2 course soon after, this time in New York, followed by his master's programme in Florida.

By now our confidence was increasing, we were doing a lot of cosmetic cases in our practices and we even became instructors for the Rosenthal programmes in the UK. We set up our own cosmetic training academy at the Hertford practice, and we were also regularly travelling to the US to attend the American Academy of Cosmetic Dentistry (AACD) meetings. At this point we began to realise the importance of occlusion and began to focus on that. At the AACD, we came across Frank Spears, who was the 'God of occlusion'! We loved his style of teaching and took all his courses. We were also introduced to laser dentistry (hard tissue and soft tissue) very early on and did a variety of courses in the US on this and now we use lasers frequently at the practice. We also took a photography course in the US and learnt from one of the best. My philosophy has always been to find the best people in their respective fields and learn from them.

Not only did we focus on clinical dentistry, we also focused on the business side of dentistry, again inspired by one of the best in the industry, Cathy Jameson. Later, we also came across Bill Blatchford, who is the number one dental coach in the US. We made a massive financial investment to take part in his one-year coaching programme, but it was worth every penny.

We also learnt the importance of marketing ourselves, including newspaper and magazine articles, being featured in three series of the *Extreme Makeover UK* television programme and a segment on *This Morning* as well as the television series *Body Shockers.* I also featured in *The Only Way Is Essex,* and on *Channel 5 News.*

At this point we found running the three practices alongside teaching too much so we decided to consolidate and initially sold the Barnet practice, followed by the Hornchurch practice about ten years ago.

A few years after selling the Hornchurch practice, Rahul and I decided amicably to end the partnership and Rahul bought my share of the Hertford practice and continued there. This was a tough time for me as I needed to find a new start and it was made harder by the fact that the UK was in a recession. To find the type of cosmetic job I wanted was very difficult. Eventually I was given the opportunity to become the lead cosmetic dentist for a chain of practices in West London. Although I was grateful for the opportunity, I knew I wanted to work for myself again and was looking for a new opportunity ... my reincarnation was about to begin!

It was at this time my family and I moved to Buckhurst Hill for schooling reasons and instinctively I knew the area had great potential. I decided to focus on setting up a new practice in the area.

My father and I drove around the area looking for properties; we had no luck until right at the end of the day, we came across a house for sale in Chigwell, in a great location. We went to view the property and it just felt right and we even got an offer accepted for the property prior to getting planning permission. It was a big gamble, but we eventually got the planning in June 2010. Despite the fact the potential practice was currently a house and the rest of the street was residential, I kept on remaining positive during the planning and believed we would eventually get approval.

For the next few months, I focused on designing the practice, building the practice, recruiting the perfect team, and setting up systems for the practice, as well as marketing, getting ready for the launch. I had to make sure I got everything right and wanted to create my dream environment, a spa-like practice offering the latest technologies. We had to make a massive investment of £1.3 million to achieve this, along with the support of my father and wife Jyoti, but I had great belief that the practice would do well so did not hesitate at the investment. A few weeks after opening, we had a launch party and over 200 people came! The practice opened in January 2011 and has been busy ever since and seven years on we are growing at the rate of 10-15% each year. We have a fantastic team with a strong focus on customer service and between us we provide the highest level of cosmetic dentistry, implants, general dentistry, laser dentistry, fibre dentistry, facial aesthetics and orthodontics in a spa-like environment. Our philosophy is to go out of our way to help our patients.

A couple of years after setting up and growing the Chigwell practice, I decided to get back to my other passion of teaching and began setting up my own training academy. I currently offer a comprehensive 8-day hands-on cosmetic/occlusion/restorative course, a one-day course called Achieving Success in Private Dentistry, and a 3-day Live Smile Makeover course.

I continue to work clinically at my practice, alongside the teaching, and am very passionate about what I do. Although I love dentistry, for me the most important aspect of life is achieving a perfect work/life balance. I love to spend time with my family, travel, play golf, tennis and spend time working on my spiritual development. I am grateful that the new start I had to make has made me even stronger and better, and I am very content in my life.

Another passion of mine is charitable work and I am heavily involved with a charity called Food For Life Vrindavan (www.fflv.org), which aims to deliver food and education to young deprived girls in India.

What is success?

Success to me is feeling happiness from within, finding your purpose in life and making a contribution to the world. My motto is "Change people's lives and make them smile," and my favourite saying is "Live the moment..."

Top tips for success

Create a clear vision and set written goals.

Focus on what you are good at and become a master at that.

Learn from the best.

No Limits

Dr Nilesh R Parmar

BDS (Lond) MSc (ProsthDent) MSc (ImpDent) Cert.Ortho MFGDP (UK) MBA

Dr Nilesh Parmar qualified in 2004 from Queen Mary's Dental School. Following this, he gained a master's degree in Prosthetic Dentistry from the Eastman Dental Institute and a master's degree in Clinical Implantology from King's College London. More recently he has completed an MBA at Imperial College, London. His main area of interest is in dental implants and he runs a successful seven-surgery practice in Southend. Over the years Nilesh has achieved many awards including Young Dentist of the Year at the 2014 Dental Awards and he has been voted in Dentistry's Top 50.

Nilesh lectures extensively, both nationally and internationally. A prolific writer, Nilesh has a regular column in the *Dental Probe Journal* and is a regular contributor to several dental publications. He runs a dental events company, a 7-surgery practice and a racing team.

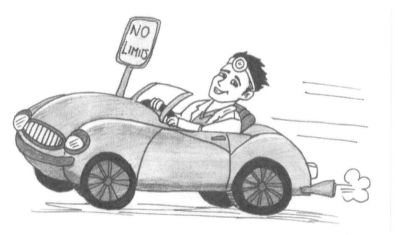

My journey into dentistry started when I was a teenager working on Saturday mornings at my dad's dental practice, sorting out orthodontic models, helping out developing X-rays in the dark room, and attempting dental nursing – which I was hopeless at! I even spent time

on reception and eventually learnt all the NHS codes during my time there.

Despite an enjoyable time at my dad's practice, I really wanted to become a surgeon, which was inspired by my love of the American television series ER. After a long time deliberating between medicine and dentistry, I finally decided to apply for dentistry, as I already had gained so much experience and did not want to do the on calls and long hours associated with medicine.

As a teenager I had a bad stammer and was a pretty reclusive individual; I had poor social skills which prevented me from talking to pretty girls! On top of this I was a very average student and only achieved average grades during my A-level mock exams. As a result of this, my teachers predicted A-level grades for me which would not be sufficient to get a place at dental school. This was a massive knock and resulted in me getting no interviews or offers to any dental schools. Rather than getting down and depressed about this, I made a choice to put in the hard work and study like never before to get the best A-level results I could. The hard work paid off and I got much better A-level grades than I was predicted but still had the dilemma of no dental school offer.

As soon as I got my results I was on the phone to go through clearing and try to get an offer and after an agonising wait on hold, I was offered a place at Queen Mary's Dental School. Hard work and sheer determination had paid off!

I started dental school in 1999 with my stammer but amazingly just seemed to lose it completely overnight! The confidence of believing in myself and getting into dental school improved my social skills and eradicated my stammer.

During my time at dental school I did not enjoy the course. I hated the systems in place and how long it took to see patients. I even started to not to turn up to clinics but in 2004 I managed to qualify, scraping through by doing the absolute bare minimum.

Soon after, another knock down came as I couldn't get a VT position locally. Yet again I was faced with more rejections. I finally managed to get a place in North Essex, which was a long commute.

Since I had done so little clinical work I really struggled during my

VT year, particularly with oral surgery. I decided I had to do something about this and so used to go every Saturday to my dad's practice to learn to take teeth out. Some mornings I struggled to barely see one patient and take a tooth out! After a while something clicked and I became more confident in my clinical ability.

During my VT year I was not liked by the other VT trainers as I was driving a brand new Porsche 911, which I had purchased soon after qualifying from profits I had made in the stock market, using my student loan as capital (investing in the dot com boom paid off!). The dislike I experienced taught me an important lesson: the more successful you are, the more people will hold it against you. I never forgot that.

Another memorable moment was during a talk by Raj Rattan at a VT study weekend. Raj asked how much the audience wanted to earn in ten years' time. He started at £50,000 per year and gradually increased the amount and as the amount increased the number of hands went down. When he reached £250,000, my hand was the only one left up. At that point he approached me and asked what figure he had to say for me to put my hand down. "£500,000!" I said. Everyone laughed – except for Raj, who said because I had the self-belief to earn that, I would be the only one in the room to do it. To this day I really value that moment. Self-belief is very important, but we all need someone to believe in us; it helps to get the process going.

Following my VT year, I went to work as an SHO at Guy's Hospital and King's College Hospital, under the guidance of Martin Kelleher. It was during this time I really began to like dentistry, in particular implant dentistry. The mentorship of Mr K was excellent, and he nurtured my ambition and helped me develop my clinical skill set. If it wasn't for that year as an SHO I would not have pursued any post graduate education.

After this, I applied for a max-fax SHO job in Basildon Hospital. I was confident I would get the position as I knew many of the staff who worked there, the interview went well but I still got another rejection. Yet another knock down and to this day I don't know the reason behind it.

I was upset and went back to speak to Mr K, who advised me to focus on postgraduate training rather than another SHO post, so I began looking into the MSc Implant course at The Eastman Dental Institute. Unfortunately, the course was fully booked and the only course they had available was an MSc Prosthetic course. My immediate thought was, "Not more dentures!" But after some deliberation I decided to do the prosthetic course; the least sexy course going!

To my surprise the year-long course was very intense and very hard but interesting at the same time. The Eastman really was a hardcore dental army camp. I was getting there at 8am and staying until 9pm most days. On top of this I was working on the weekends at my dad's practice to help with finances plus also doing lab work on the weekends for the course. It was a very difficult year, but I somehow got through it and gained my first postgraduate degree. I now love making dentures!

I still wanted to do implant training and luckily Guy's Hospital ran a part time two-year MSc programme. The course only took on four candidates and was very competitive. I applied for the course and managed to get an interview. Luckily, I knew both interviewers and was confident that I would get on the course. To my surprise I got a rejection the day after the interview and was told I made it to number five and missed out on the top four as I was too inexperienced. Yet another knock down! Luckily, three weeks before the course started I got a call to say that one of the delegates could no longer make it so I managed to finally get onto an Implant MSc programme!

The implant programme was amazing – it changed my life. My implant journey had finally begun and has accelerated ever since, leading to today, where I currently place on average over 300 implants a year and run a comprehensive implant course (Implant Academy) with Avik Dandapat. I cannot explain how satisfying it is to work hard at becoming good at something, executing it, and seeing for yourself that you really can do it. It's not ego, but satisfaction.

Soon after the implant programme I became a partner in my dad's practice and completed a certificate in orthodontics at Warwick University. I wasn't as keen on ortho compared to implants, and felt the teaching was a bit basic compared to what I was used to. Nevertheless, I did gain an insight into another area of dentistry.

I have always had a keen interest in business and, following a trip to a business fair, I decided to apply for an MBA at Imperial College London in 2014. The MBA was a truly amazing course but super difficult, the knowledge I gained was invaluable and I felt it rounded me off as a person. I learnt that being a dentist is great, but being an entrepreneur is even better!

On the back of my MBA I had the confidence to set up my own company, NP Racing and Promotions, which combines my passions for car racing and dentistry. I am a big believer in multiple sources of income and have a better ability to do this following my MBA.

Charity to me is equally as important as making money and this has driven me to organise an annual Christmas party known as the ICE WHITE PARTY, with all proceeds going to different charities every year. We have managed to raise over £40,000 so far. I am also looking into setting up my own charitable organisation.

I currently spend the majority of my time at my practice in Southend, which we recently expanded and refurbished to a very high spec. We even won an award for the most high-tech practice in the UK! My inspiration in design was to think if Tony Stark (Iron Man) was to build a dental practice, what would it look like? I also work one day a week in London at a private practice, solely placing implants. On top of this I am busy with training courses, lecturing, social media, charitable events and car racing!

My advice to any young dentist is work hard. The BDS is just the beginning. I have worked seven-day weeks for as long as I can remember, and I never fully shut off. Holidays need to be earned, not expected, and your time should always be used effectively. Find a hobby, something that you enjoy and have that as your release. Excel in what you do and enjoy your successes! There is nothing wrong with being successful.

What is success?

To me, success is to maximise and live up to your potential.

Top tips for success

Always have your foot on the accelerator and keep moving forward.

Pushing the Boundary

Dr Amit Patel
BDS MSc MClinDent FDS RCSEd MRD RCSEng

Dr Amit Patel graduated from the University of Liverpool in 1997. He then went on to complete a four-year specialist training programme in periodontics at Guy's, King's & St Thomas' (GKT) Dental Institute. His special interests are dental implants, regenerative and aesthetic periodontics. Amit has his own specialist private practice, Birmingham Dental Specialists, based in the heart of Birmingham. He also teaches and lectures both in the UK and internationally.

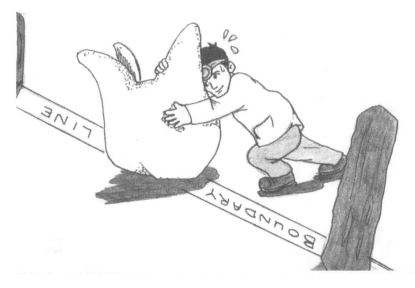

Throughout school I was never too interested in studying. My plan was to leave school at the age of 16 and join the forces or become a plumber, but I stayed on as my friends were staying to do their A-levels. During this time my teachers suggested I should apply for dentistry and without much thought I decided I would! I had done no research or planning into a career in dentistry but decided to give it a go. With a poor interview technique, getting a place at dental school became a challenge in itself, but after many rejections my final interview at the University of Liverpool resulted in an offer.

Growing up in London and having to move to Liverpool was a big culture shock. Liverpool was definitely not like London but there were also lots of positives: the people were so friendly, the city was amazing and the student union was one of the biggest in Europe at that time. I did enjoy Liverpool, but I realised within my first term that I didn't want to be a dentist for the rest of my life! Since I was enjoying the university lifestyle I decided to carry on with the course, barely just scraping through without much interest in the subject. This began to change in the fourth year when I went to the Maxillofacial Department and saw head and neck dissections; it was the first time my interest was piqued and I became fascinated in the course. I began to spend time with the maxillo-facial surgeons and they allowed me to come in to theatre and help hands on with major surgical procedures. After this experience I was convinced that I wanted to become a maxillo-facial surgeon.

After graduating I stayed on at the university and became a house officer and then senior house officer and acquired my MFDS. Following this, I did my vocational training and applied for medicine. Leeds University gave me an offer on their shortened course, which I was delighted with. Before starting medicine, I did a max-fax job at University College London, which had a big impact on me. I met some really unhappy and stressed-out surgeons who seemed to have been chewed up in the system and at that point I decided a career in max-fax was not for me. There was no guarantee I was going to be working in an exceptional unit and the NHS was changing with regards to training.

I wasn't sure of the next direction I would take but remembered from my year as a VT meeting some very enthusiastic specialists, one a periodontist and one an endodontist. After going out for dinner with these two specialists I decided I wanted to specialise in periodontics. I applied for the speciality programme at GKT and after another exceptionally poor interview I somehow managed to gain a place in the programme. I started the programme in 2001 and soon got bored of it! I was beginning to think I had made the wrong decision and should have done medicine instead. Luckily for me, one of my lecturers on the programme was a periodontist called Dr Alan Sidi. He is a brilliant individual, very enthusiastic and performed the most amazing surgery. He inspired me and showed me what I could be; this immediately changed my focus away from medicine and back to periodontics. Four years later I gained my MSc in periodontology and a MClinDent in periodontics, followed by my exit exam, which I sat at the Royal College of Surgeons of England. This led to me becoming a specialist periodontist.

Once I became a specialist I went looking for work – which was harder to find than I thought. When I became a specialist I thought I was at the top of the pyramid, but I soon realised specialists are at the bottom of the pyramid as we rely on general dental practitioners who are at the top to refer to us. I did manage to find work, travelling all over the country to many top practices based in Manchester, London and Bath. During this time I learnt the importance of building relationships and rapport with referring dentists and with patients. At the Bath practice my journey into implants accelerated; I was able to observe many implant placements and also started routinely placing implants myself. I had the opportunity to see and learn how to push the limits of implants.

My thirst for knowledge did not stop after I became a specialist; in fact, I was even hungrier to learn the latest and most advanced techniques and technology in the field of implants and periodontics. This led me to travel all over the world and attend the most amazing courses and seminars with the most forward thinking individuals. I even got involved in research at Harvard University and at the University of Milan. I loved to push the boundaries in periodontics and implant dentistry using all the techniques I learnt abroad, and still follow the same philosophy to this day.

In 2007 I moved to Birmingham as my girlfriend, who is an anaesthetist, was training there. I found work close by and flew once a week to Belfast to place implants and do periodontics there. I also worked as an associate specialist for Professor Iain Chapple, an amazing clinician who let me practice all the latest techniques I had learnt from abroad; he let me push the boundaries and never questioned my treatment techniques. From this, new opportunities arose for me. Professor Chapple put my name forward to lecture instead of him. I was invited to lecture across the UK, Sweden, Poland and many other countries. I was also invited to start publishing my work in a variety of journals and books.

During this time, I also decided to take the plunge and set up my own referral practice in Birmingham. The practice continues to do well as over time I have slowly built up my reputation with referring dentists.

What is success?

Success is not competing with anyone else – only with yourself. Our profession can be very competitive, but I have always just focused on myself to be the best I can be and to continually learn and better myself. I see myself as an average periodontist; I hope one day I will be a good periodontist.

Top tips for success

To this day I have no regrets about not doing medicine. What I have learnt over the last 20 years and what keeps me going is the enjoyment I get from talking to patients, meeting new people, making them feel special and trying my best to help them. This is the best tip I can give anyone.

Another tip of mine relates to the use of social media in dentistry. Unfortunately, some of the comments and feedback on social media can be very negative and critical; my advice is to not take any of these comments seriously.

The Calling

Melonie Prebble
RDH RDT

Melonie Prebble qualified in Dental Hygiene and Therapy in 1995 at the Royal London. Mel is a dental hygienist and therapist with over 20 years in the industry where she has worked in a range of clinical settings. In addition to her clinical work she is interested in business development skills and is a qualified Master Neuro Linguistic Programming coach. She is a regular contributor to the dental industry, attending events as a speaker, contributing to journals and sitting on dental award judging panels.

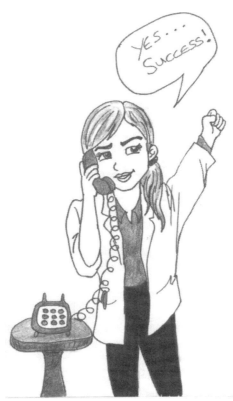

At school I wanted to be something different every day; I never really knew what to do when I was older. At the age of 15 I decided I needed to make some money so I found a Saturday job dental nursing at a local dental practice. I didn't have much of a clue what I was doing but I knew I really liked it!

After my O-Levels I didn't believe I would be able to do well in my A-levels so, since I liked dental nursing, I decided instead to take my nursing qualifications alongside working at the same practice. After qualifying I stayed on at the practice nursing, but soon realised I wanted to do more and get more involved with treating the patients. A friend of mine suggested looking into dental hygiene and therapy.

I decided to apply to the Royal London, who at that time were the only institute offering training in Hygiene and Therapy. I soon got a rejection letter. At that point I made a decision not to accept the rejection. I picked up the phone, called the institute and managed to convince them, so much so that they offered me an interview.

After the interview I won my place and off I went to London. I found the course very challenging, especially academically, but I put in the hard work, spending most evenings in the library studying. The great thing about the course was that it was integrated with the dental course, allowing me to gain a very broad knowledge of dentistry.

After qualifying I soon found hygiene work in a variety of different practices during the week. During that time there was not much demand for therapy work so I focused on hygiene treatments. I didn't enjoy general practice; I found a massive difference in what I had learned to what I was allowed to do in general practice and thought I had made the worst mistake of my life!

I began looking for a new job, hoping to find a practice that allowed me to work the way I was trained to, and luckily managed to find a job in a practice in Watford, working as a tag team with an oral health educator. This job allowed me to realise the potential I had in my career and in myself. The practice was very innovative and forward thinking and invested a great deal in further training.

I began to attend a variety of different courses, not just in the UK but all over the world. From my experiences abroad, I soon realised how under-used hygienists and therapists were in the UK. At the practice we implemented many of the systems I had learned abroad, including the hygienist-led exams. Over the years I have evolved these systems to make them work for me in my practices.

On my travels in the United States I was introduced to a company that delivers practice management consultancy and was given the opportunity to work with this US-based company but in the UK, delivering practice management consultancy, which I did for about five years. The company was set up by a hygienist with an ethos of improving practices through utilising the hygienist more effectively and appropriately.

I made it my point not only to attend hygiene/therapy courses but also courses aimed at dentists, to further my knowledge of what is possible. This included cosmetic courses, implant courses and occlusion courses. I also wanted to improve my non-clinical 'soft' skills, which to me are equally as important as the clinical skills, so I embarked on a journey to improve my communication skills which eventually led me to become a Master in Neuro Linguistic Programming. Becoming a Master NLP practitioner has been life-changing and has paid dividends in my work.

In the mid-2000s, as soon as regulations changed allowing therapists to work in general practice, I was determined to start working as a therapist as well as a hygienist and went through the process of re-skilling myself as I had lost a lot of these skills following university. During this time, I also decided to set up my own course programme as I wanted to impart all the knowledge I had gained. It was a four-day programme including clinical and non-clinical topics aimed at hygienists/therapists.

In 2008 I decided to start a family and took a small break from clinical work. However, I was still delivering practice management consultancy and my training courses during my pregnancy and even after whilst I was breastfeeding! Since I loved my clinical work so much I only took off three months but when I returned I decided to move on from my current practices for a new start elsewhere. This included starting in a practice in St John's Wood, which had never had a hygienist before. This was like Nirvana for me, as I could set up how I wanted to work from the get go. At the same time, I took on a similar job at a private practice in Welwyn, which again allowed me to put systems in place.

I continue to work in both these practices but also am involved with two dental companies, Dentsply Sirona and Philips, as a key opinion leader, delivering education and training.

My relationship with Dentsply Sirona flourished after being invited to go to Berlin in 2012 for one of their Ultrasonic Sonic programmes. Since then I work with the company as a key opinion leader working at exhibitions, sometimes as a keynote speaker or on the stand, plus training with their sales team and working with their PR team. I joined the team at Philips more recently in 2016, after being approached by them.

What is success?

Success equals happiness; to me, it is not measured by anything tangible, but is about enjoying doing what I want to do.

Top tips for success

There is no such thing as failure, only feedback.

There is not always a wrong or right, as long as you are confident in yourself that you are doing the right thing.

Be curious and ask why.

Leave work at work and enjoy yourself!

A Series of Fortunate Events

Dr Tif Qureshi
BDS

Dr Tif Qureshi qualified from King's College London in 1992. Tif has a special interest in orthodontics and minimally invasive dentistry. He was the first dentist in the UK to pioneer and develop the Inman Aligner concept and its protocols. He is the clinical director of the IAS Academy, an international faculty that provides mentored education for general dentists on a pathway from simple to comprehensive orthodontics. Tif also pioneered the concept of alignment, bleaching and bonding to create the perfect smile in a more minimally invasive but also very functional way. He is an experienced teacher in the Dahl concept. Tif lectures nationally and internationally and has had many articles published on all these subjects. He is also a past president of the British Academy of Cosmetic Dentistry (BACD).

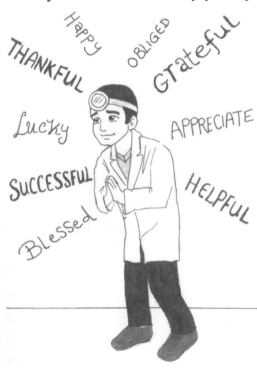

My childhood was spent in Kent and I grew up in a family of doctors; both my mother and father were GPs, which gave me only two choices for my future career: medicine or dentistry! Asian culture was always focused on becoming a professional because in those days it was considered a 'safe choice' and I was reasonably happy to be gently pushed in that direction.

I was thrilled when I got into dental school but had a shock fairly soon after the second year when I realised I wasn't enjoying it at all. Despite this, I managed to get through it and qualified in 1992 relatively unscathed. There were some great clinicians teaching at King's who made it worthwhile.

After graduating, I moved back home to Rochester and completed my vocational training (VT) at a practice nearby. I began to enjoy dentistry slightly more during my VT year and had some great mentors who taught me so much, not just clinically but also in patient communication. At this point I still wasn't sure about a long-term career in dentistry and began doubting if I had chosen the right course.

Despite my reservations, following my VT year I began working as an associate in an NHS practice in Sidcup. I had no idea this would be where I would be doing what I am now 26 years later.

The first four years at the practice were extremely tough and I very quickly really started to dislike dentistry. It wasn't the actual work, it was the fact that patients seemed naturally suspicious of dentists generally and seemed to automatically assume dentists were out to rip them off. Typically, the comment "Don't be offended but I hate dentists" would often ruin my day. I found these comments painful, when I felt I was only trying to do the right thing. I even started the process of a career change to become a computer games tester/programmer!

However, I decided to buy an Intra Oral Camera – it was one of the first in the UK (22 years ago) – and this literally changed everything overnight. Patients could see everything and became far more educated and understanding of what we needed to do. Quite why so few dentists use them in everyday practice in 2018 I have no idea- this tool has been the most important in my whole career. From that day forward, I really started to enjoy treating people. I took some courses in restorative dentistry (Mike Wise was brilliant), composites and photography. Attending these courses ignited a new sense of excitement for dentistry.

A big turning point in my career came in the early 2000s when I was involved in the process of setting up the BACD. I also met Tim Bradstock-Smith, who later became a business partner and friend. Over time I became more involved in aesthetic dentistry, attending many courses on veneers. Some of them were very controversial to me even back then, but they certainly taught me a lot about the kind of dentistry I did and didn't want to do. It was the teaching of minimally invasive dentistry from people such as Sverker Toreskog, Bjorn Zachrisson (a legendary orthodontist) and Pascal Magne which would become very influential in my career; their courses and lectures were mind altering!

I put what I learnt into practice and began completing many veneer cases. However, I always found I had a greater affinity and love for composites and preferred the minimally invasive approach rather than cutting teeth down. A real issue was the fact that in the late nineties, Anterior Alignment Orthodontics did not really exist so veneers were a more popular choice for patients, who commonly refused the comprehensive orthodontic sole option they were offered. I began offering simple orthodontics using removable appliances which I had briefly learnt about at dental school. It was interesting how simple minor movements could make such a difference to a patient's perception.

The really big turning point came in about 2004. As an American Academy of Cosmetic Dentistry (AACD) member I came across an interesting article in the AACD journal about the Inman aligner. I contacted the lab that was making these aligners and discussed the possibility of sending some of my cases to them in the US. Don Inman, the technician who invented the aligner, gave me the opportunity to work a few of my cases with him and I was surprised and amazed by the results I was getting. Bjorn Zachrisson helped and mentored me greatly when I first started with the Inman aligner. Spurred on by these consistent great results, I began to start lecturing on the Inman aligner at various BACD study clubs and eventually at many conferences. Following the BACD conference there was a huge demand from members wanting to know how to provide this simple alignment treatment instead of veneer-based dentistry, so we decided to run a simple course. I did this with James Russell and Tim Bradstock-Smith.

Don Inman realised I could make this aligner do a lot more than he ever imagined so he gave us the global rights to train dentists on to use the appliance. The courses in the UK proved very popular and soon I was being invited to other parts of the world to lecture and run courses on the Inman aligner, including Europe, Australia, the Middle East and the USA.

We started using more forms of orthodontic aligners, including clear aligners and fixed braces, and so began the process of setting up the IAS Academy in about 2012. The IAS Academy continues to grow worldwide, and we have courses and labs set up in most of the countries we operate from. Anoop Maini soon joined the IAS Academy to teach fixed orthodontics, followed by Professor Ross Hobson who joined the Academy to help with setting high standards of case selection, consent, record keeping and treatment planning. Our goal became to never teach a 'system' but to teach appropriate restoratively-focused orthodontics.

Another concept that I am passionate about is our ortho/ restorative programme. This covers the importance of occlusion, function and orthodontic planning which respects, improves and maintains the envelope of function. I also love teaching the Dahl Principle as part of this thinking. I was lucky enough to be taught the Dahl Principle by Martin Kelleher at dental school. These principles have allowed me to treat patients successfully over many decades and I have developed a methodology with Dahl that I believe is one of the most useful tools in dentistry, one that is still massively underused and could change the way every dentist in the world approaches wear cases early on.

In fact, IAS is not an 'ortho academy' at all, it is uniquely an academy of ortho/ restorative/ functional and minimally invasive dentistry – and I believe there is nothing else like it.

Looking back at my career, I am grateful for the opportunities I had including being president of the BACD (interestingly, I was the first

BACD president that had to be voted in). Currently I'm a director of the IAS Academy; however, I still like to tell people I am just a BDS. My greatest accomplishment and most important learning experience has been working in the same practice for over twenty-six years, photographing all my work, seeing and learning from all my failures and successes. I have learnt more from my own cases than any course I have ever been on.

I still work clinically at our practice in Kent and still love clinical dentistry. The rest of the time I am busy teaching, mentoring and lecturing all over the world. Teaching has become a real passion of mine and I want to help as many dentists as I can to do the type of dentistry I do and make as much of a difference as I can in our profession.

What is success?

Success to me is not about money, notoriety or awards. To me it is about making a difference in the profession.

Top tips for success

Just follow the Golden Rule and treat people how you would want to be treated yourself.

Photograph all your cases – or you are missing out on the biggest learning experience in dentistry.

The Year of Change

Dr Alun Rees
BDS

Dr Alun Rees qualified from Newcastle University in 1978. He started his career as an oral surgery resident, eventually becoming a multiple practice owner. A career change in 2004 led him to follow his passion and become The Dental Business Coach. He now spends his time as a coach, helping dentists improve their working lives and helping them achieve the rewards their hard work and dedication deserve.

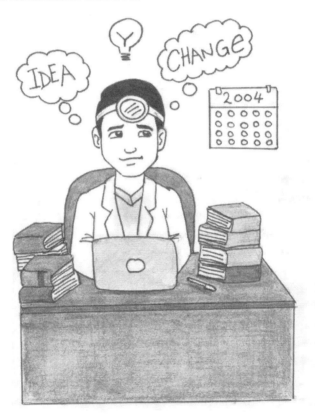

Brought up in South Wales, my first experience of dentistry was not a pleasant one. At the age of six I underwent extraction of multiple teeth under general anaesthetic, which made me very phobic of dentists.

Eventually my mother took me to a lady dentist in the suburbs of Cardiff where we lived; this dentist was absolutely wonderful and slowly, over time, managed to alleviate my fear of dentistry. From these experiences in my childhood, I knew very early on from about the age of twelve that I wanted to do nothing else but become a dentist. The way that this dentist had helped me was something that I wanted to do for others.

Eventually I made it to dental school at Newcastle and had five fantastic years. I wasn't the most dedicated academically, but I had a great time! When I qualified I didn't want to go straight into general practice; I had an interest in treating trauma, so I took up an oral surgery residency at the Royal London Hospital. This was an incredibly intense, amazing and informative time for me. I then went to Kettering Hospital where I got a lot of hands-on experience, followed by a stint at University Hospital of South Manchester in Withington. It was here where I decided I didn't want to do oral surgery as a career. I got what I needed from these experiences and became confident in dealing with surgical dentistry.

After hospital I spent about seven years as an associate in a variety of practices in and around Peterborough developing my philosophy of dentistry. I wanted to work in a way that put the patient's health at the centre of everything. In 1998 I decided to take the plunge and start my own practice in Gloucester. The practice was set up as a cold squat and did well, so well that 15 months later I decided to start another practice. This coincided with a downturn in the economy, significant increases in interest rates and the failure of my first marriage. Obviously this was a difficult time, leaving me no choice but to redouble my efforts to make my business successful, which is what I did, and I started looking at the business side of dentistry more. By 1993, business was going well: one practice was closed, I had re-married and life was good. My wife was a dental hygienist and together we built our successful practice, where prevention and health were cornerstones. In the wake of the 1992 fee costs we had significantly reduced our reliance on the NHS. During this time, I invested in postgraduate training to up my skills, including restorative courses, a fresh focus on perio and I also did some orthodontic training. On every measure the business was successful, we were profitable and there was a plentiful supply of new patients coming from personal recommendation, but in 2004 I decided I had hit a ceiling! I had one of those light bulb moments and knew that I didn't want to practice dentistry for the rest of my life. I realised that the clinical part of dentistry no longer satisfied me and once I realised this, there was no turning back. I sold the practice in 2005.

The next five years were a mix of locum jobs in a variety of different practices, some nice, some not so nice and growing my non-clinical career. Earlier on I had studied the MBA course at the Open University and this helped me to develop my interest in the business side of dentistry. Having worked in the past with different dental coaches I decided to do my coaching training and this allowed me to start helping some of the practices where I was a locum. Gradually I become more and more involved in helping the development of practices and any dependence on clinical work had disappeared by 2011.

At the end of 2013 we burned our bridges: I made the decision to come off the General Dental Council register and we moved from our home in Gloucestershire to what had been our holiday home in South West Ireland. From here I continue to grow The Dental Business Coach. My work takes me all over, and beyond, the UK and Ireland, helping dental business owners and their teams.

Some clients want my services as a one off, an intensive day of analysis, ideas and suggestions for change and improvements; others opt for a more long-term relationship where I can help them achieve change and make progress in a continuous way.

What is success?

There are lots of definitions of success but my favourite for dentists is 'Improving your condition whilst improving the condition of those around you.' Success is best shared; I believe there is plenty to go around.

Top tips for success

My first tip is a rule for life: "Set your course by the stars, not by the lights of every passing ship"; take the long view and don't be distracted by all the bright shiny objects. You are in this game of life and dentistry is a big part of it, but there is more to life. Don't get distracted by things that are not taking you in the right direction; be clear of what your aims, goals and dreams are.

For success within dentistry you must accept you are a professional. That means many things but primarily, focussing on your patients, putting them at the centre of everything that you do, discovering their needs and wants and then addressing them. Sometimes it means doing it when you don't want to. Dentistry is not an easy career, but you are fortunate to be able to do it. You must respect and earn the trust that people put in you.

Do as much learning while you can and never stop learning; getting your BDS is only the start. Once you stop learning, stop being curious, stop developing yourself, stop looking beyond where you are, then you are going backwards.

Paper Boy to Property Boy

Dr Harry Singh
BChD, MFGDP

Dr Harry Singh qualified from Leeds University in 1996. During his time as a dentist and award-winning practice owner, Harry developed a keen interest in facial aesthetics, completing over 3000 cases since 2002. He is the founder of the Botulinum Toxin Club and now regularly trains and lectures all over the UK. His main passion, however, has always been in property and now he has a property portfolio worth over seven million pounds. Harry shares his property secrets by training dentists through his Dental Property Club programme.

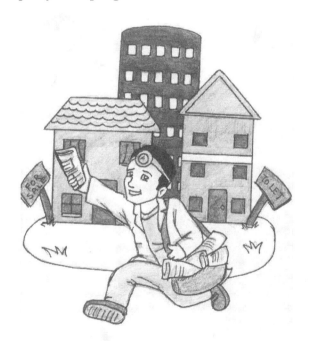

I knew from an early age I wanted to become a dentist. I enjoyed science at school and, coming from an Indian family, I was always steered towards a career in medicine or dentistry. My mother was disappointed I was contemplating dentistry, feeling that it was medicine's poorer brother! Despite my mother's reservations, after doing some work experience at a local dental practice and seeing the dentist's watch and car, I made up my mind to do dentistry! Part of the attraction to dentistry was the money so I embarked on my dental career at Leeds University. Within the first year of university I soon discovered that I was not passionate about dentistry, but I chose to stick it out as I didn't want to be a failure in my parents' eyes.

After qualifying in 1996, I followed the traditional path of vocational training, associate and then principal. I knew very early on in my career that my long-term goal was not to stay in dentistry – I did not enjoy it, I had no passion for it – and I set a definitive plan of action to accomplish this. Part of this plan was to save as much money as possible and live within my means. While my vocational trainee friends were out spending money on cars and watches I was saving up, driving a cheap car, living with my parents; all for the goal of exiting dentistry. The dental profession also allowed me to gain suitable income to follow my real passion, which was property.

My passion in property came at an early age when I was a paper boy. On a normal Sunday morning delivering newspapers, one client told me to keep his paper as he did not want it. The newspaper was the Sunday Times and it just so happened to feature the Rich List. As I was reading this article I worked out over 80% of the people featured on this list made their money either directly or indirectly from property. I thought, if that's good enough for them, then that's good enough for me!

In 2002 I set up my first squat dental practice with a friend, based in Bedfordshire. I then decided to develop my knowledge of facial aesthetics and cosmetic dentistry, which led to me attending many postgraduate courses. I found a real interest in facial aesthetics and enjoyed completing these types of cases. Facial aesthetics felt completely different to dentistry; it didn't feel like work. It was also during this time I began investing in property the traditional way.

In 2003, at a property auction, by chance I met a property guru who became my mentor on the secrets of professional property investments. Over the next two years I managed to buy and hold 27 properties and sell six properties. During this time, I was still practising dentistry and was also a vocational trainer plus I invested further in advanced facial aesthetic training.

In 2006, at the age of 34, I achieved financial freedom as a result of the passive income I was receiving from my property portfolio.

This passive income allowed me to set up another squat practice in 2007, this time in Hertfordshire. This became an award-winning practice and focused mainly on facial aesthetics. As my experience and skills in facial aesthetics grew, I was invited to write numerous articles for various professional magazines and became a speaker on facial aesthetics at dental events.

I finally decided in 2012 to give up my practice and my career in dentistry. Over the years I had many friends and colleagues who were always asking how I managed to earn enough to give up dentistry. So I decided to set up the Dental Property Club to teach my fellow colleagues the property secrets and financial education that gave me my financial freedom.

Following this I also set up the Botox Training Club (now called Botulinum Toxin Club) in 2014, after noticing that many friends and colleagues had learnt how to do facial aesthetic treatments but lacked the marketing knowledge to get clients in.

My time is now spent doing what I love, which includes spending plenty of time with my family, pursuing my hobbies and interests as well as teaching, property investing and providing facial aesthetic treatments two days a week. My week does not feel like work as I thoroughly enjoy every part of it and, due to my financial freedom, I have no pressure from my working life.

What is success?

Success is not a goal, it is a journey to continue to better yourself and develop yourself to be the best you can. It is about waking up and doing what you love, what you are good at and what pays well.

Top tips for success

Don't follow the crowd; follow your own path and your own dreams, and this will make you truly happy.

How do we become wealthy? There is a process and if followed it will lead to success. There are three levels that you will want to complete in the correct order to achieve massive wealth. Your aim is to invest in assets that will produce passive income every month, no matter what you do yourself. Once you reach each level, you will build up more passive income until you reach level three – and then you can celebrate. Initially you will have your working income too, but once your passive income takes over, you may decide either to stop working or to work only when you want to.

Level 1 – Financial Security – enough passive income to cover the bare essentials, such as food, shelter, utility bills, essential expenses like clothing, insurance, motor maintenance, etc. For most people this figure will be less that £2,000pcm.

Level 2 – Financial Independence – enough passive income to maintain your current lifestyle. For most people this will be between £2,000pcm -£5,000pcm.

Level 3 – Financial Freedom – enough passive income to live your dream lifestyle. For most people this will be £10,000pcm+.

Systems and Data Man

Dr Asif Syed
BDS

Dr Asif Syed qualified from Liverpool Dental School in 1992. Asif has always had a deep interest in figures, data and the business side of dentistry. Early in his career he developed systems and structures to grow his own revenue and his practice revenues. Operating solely by referral, he began working as a business strategist with many dental practices around the UK. He successfully develops and grows dental businesses and runs courses at the BDA for young dentists, associate dentists and practice principals.

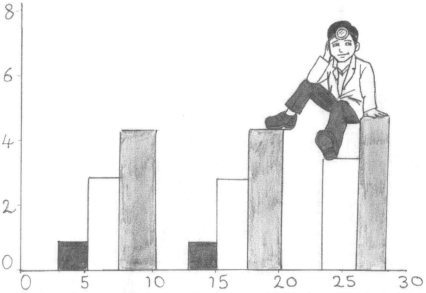

I started as an above average student in a below average school and ended up a below average student in an above average school. I had discovered all the usual distractions for a 17-year-old boy. This led to a practical implication – my school elected not to support my application to read dentistry at university. My academic statistics made grim reading: low percentile ranking in the school year, poor end of year exam performance, unimpressive mock exam results, underwhelming homework assessment, substandard predicted grades and uninspiring best-case scenarios.

Forced to consider courses I'd never heard of at universities I had no intention of attending, I decided to take a long autumnal walk through King's Heath Park, Birmingham to reconcile my situation. As a twig cracked loudly underfoot I decided to return to school with my own statistics:

- If I was 1/90 students in my year, how many hours had any one teacher spent on assessing my career choice vs the number of hours I had spent assessing my career choice?
- Number of applications supported for dentistry each year vs number of actual offer grades reached.
- My average school performance over the last 16 months vs my average school performance over the last 6 years.
- What is possible with a realistic percentage improvement vs just what the school have seen is possible over the years.

My school were impressed but unconvinced. Strangely, this no longer mattered as I had completely convinced myself.

As is likely for most people reading this book, I applied tremendous effort to reach my required grades. With grades in hand, I secured a place at dental school through the university clearing system, but with one big difference: this time my application was supported by my school.

Key learning: Everyone backs a winner. If you make an effort and look like you're heading for a win, you tend to get all the assistance you need as people have a natural inclination to associate themselves with success. If you make less effort and look like you're going to lose, you tend to get none of the assistance on offer as people have a natural inclination to distance themselves from failure.

Once at dental school, I started as a below average student but this time I stayed there too. Although I enjoyed university life and learning about dentistry, I found the course teaching largely unstructured, sometimes pointless, and nearly always political. As cliques formed and egos expanded I found my interest waned. Luckily, I found the world of work to be entirely different. As a VT I found my foundation year teaching to be highly structured, always relevant, and based on the opposite of politics, which I saw as economics. Through this lens, I gained enthusiasm for a world of work based on economics, collaboration and merit.

Returning to the dental hospital as an SHO, I was able to test this insight: if I could learn from the best to do better dentistry then I would eventually earn more in practice (economics); if I could learn to align with each individual department's agenda then I would learn more quickly (collaboration); if I could demonstrate increasing competence then they would give me more experience (merit).

Applying the world of work to a hospital environment resulted in one of my happiest years as a dentist, and the irony did not escape me: it was a return to a teaching facility I had previously disliked. This gifted me one of my best career learnings.

Key learning: Your environment is the best predictor of your performance. Take full responsibility to find, form, craft or create any given environment to get the best out of yourself.

Having completed my tenure as an SHO it was time to work as an associate with the likeable Mr Sharma. My first weeks in general dental practice were a shamble of missed bookings, random emergencies, late nurses, lost notes and insufficient materials – there was much to put right. I had to 'create the environment'. Working three days a week allowed me to test and develop systems and use statistics to measure their efficacy. Within a few months working part time, I was earning more than my full-time principal. Soon, Mr Sharma's curiosity was raised so we implemented the same systems in his surgery, measured the same metrics and achieved the same result. We planned for a practice expansion and refurbishment and all with smiles on our faces as we had an excellent relationship.

Later, my friends in London requested similar assistance so I happily relocated and refined some of the systems and metrics for them, and for my principal in his London practice too. As we achieved consistent results, expansion and refurbishment soon followed and drew attention from other practices. I'd somehow acquired a reputation for dental business management.

This attention led to another crossroads: do I continue working as a dentist or do I pursue this unknown path into dental business management? Another walk and several twigs later I arrived at a conclusion and another career lesson:

Key learning: Better to be at the bottom of a ladder you want to get to the top of than halfway up a ladder you don't.

With this decision made, events unfolded quite quickly. My practice happily supported me to take a six-month complete clinical sabbatical to work on several important dental business management projects. As word of mouth referral grew, six months turned into one year, which turned into three years until one day, over five years later, I accepted I was no longer a clinician.

Once my client list was full, I started running courses, and when our courses snowballed, we started building a team.

Like all of us, I am still climbing the ladder. Occasionally I slide down a snake, but I feel privileged every day to work on things I enjoy with people I love. If in some small way my thoughts can assist you I would summarise them here:

Key learning summary:
- Everyone backs a winner.
- Create the environment.
- Tread lightly: people are more fragile than you can possibly imagine.
- Pay attention to things you like, not things you don't.
- When presented with a new opportunity, give more than you take.
- Better to be at the bottom of a ladder you want to get to the top of than halfway up a ladder you don't.
- To be good at something important takes five years and to build a reputation for it takes ten years.

What is success?

Lifestyle. Lifestyle means you can happily succeed across multiple areas of life simultaneously, such as growing a business, raising a family, buying a house, travelling, staying fit, maintaining friendships and taking time to recharge. This is fiendishly difficult as a deficiency in one area (e.g. fitness) is not compensated for by performance in another (e.g. high earnings). Money itself won't create this balance; it only makes it easier. However, achieving lifestyle means you can enjoy every day instead of slaving away for some distant fantasy situation. This is priceless.

Top tips for success:

Here is a quote that has stayed with me for some time: "Any paid work you don't enjoy is the same as prostitution" – Morgan Freeman.

The joy of finding engaging work removes the burden of the daily grind. It is a prize worth seeking at the earliest opportunity. It will rarely fall in your lap so if you have to put in a little effort to find it, that's okay.

The Health Cultivator

Dr Andrew Toy
BDS M.Med.Sci. MFGDP (UK)

Dr Andrew Toy qualified from Bristol University in 1980. Andy has a special interest in orthodontics and is a platinum Invisalign provider, as well as a clinical lecturer on Invisalign for Align Tech UK. Andy's main passion is providing relationship-based dentistry, which is a philosophy he gained through visiting the Pankey Institute in the 1980s. He also became the first UK GDP to gain a master's degree in Clinical Education in 1999. During his career Andy has been involved in teaching, lecturing and research projects and he also set up The Dental Business Academy, an online school providing qualifications for dental team members.

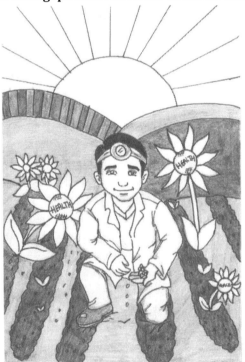

I grew up in the Welsh valleys in the 60s during a period of high unemployment. The school I attended always pushed us towards becoming a professional, as you were guaranteed a job. I enjoyed learning about science so focused on a career in dentistry, pharmacy or medicine. I liked the idea of working in a team and that attracted me more towards a career in dentistry. Also, I wasn't very dextrous and liked the challenge of learning to work with my hands!

In 1976 I started at Bristol University. Coming from the valleys into a big city opened my eyes to a new incredible world! I loved the city but unfortunately grew to hate dentistry during my time there. I struggled on through the course and just about qualified in 1980, scraping through a pass/fail viva! Whilst I hated dentistry, I also had a big overdraft that needed to be paid off.

My job hunt began, and I stumbled on an advertisement for a job in Louth, Lincolnshire. My attention was drawn to the statement: 'I will teach you general practice.' My plan was to land the job, pay off my overdraft and then go back to university to study something else! I was invited to visit this practice, which was owned by Bob Borrill and situated in a beautiful market town. The practice immediately impressed me. It was a very modern and happy place with oral health educators and an extended duties team. It was very different to the average dental practice.

Bob explained that his practice was following a philosophy of 'Health Cultivation'. He aimed to reduce dental disease in his community by building relationships with families of patients and guiding them towards a healthy lifestyle. At this point a light bulb went on in my head: this is why I wanted to be a dentist. It was a far cry from the image of practice I had learned at university, which was all 'blood, sweat and pus!' and the teaching at university, which was drill and fill. Bob showed me how we could improve people's health by doing something positive. From this point on I couldn't wait to be a dentist!

Bob offered me a position, but he confessed it wouldn't be in the beautiful village of Louth but instead, in his new practice in Grimsby – not so beautiful! From January 1981 he would mentor me once a week in Health Cultivation and all aspects of general dentistry. This was vocational training before it existed.

I now loved my dentistry and attended a lot of weekend courses. On one of those courses a senior colleague advised me to go and learn occlusion at the Pankey Institute. So, in 1982, I headed to the institute in Miami. When I got there I soon realised there was more to this institute than just occlusion. The institute had its own philosophy of comprehensive, relationship-based care. Another cornerstone of the Pankey philosophy was the importance of your own personal growth and work-life balance. This experience provided a sort of curriculum for my future 'life in dentistry'. It was undoubtedly the best money I ever spent on dental education – and I have spent a lot!

In 1983 it was time for me to move on from Bob's practice, as his son was about to qualify. I didn't want an associate job to 'drill, fill and bill'. I wanted to be a Health Cultivator. This sort of post was impossible to find. My only option was to set up a squat NHS practice.

I decided to focus on the Midlands area as it was halfway between Grimsby and Wales, plus on weekends I always found myself in Leicester with friends having my favourite food – curry! I chose Loughborough as it was growing rapidly with new houses and a new shopping centre and there was a need for a dentist in the area. The only issue was difficulty was finding a decent building to convert. However, there was some land available so, with the help of my brother (an architect), I decided to build a practice – from scratch. This was like a dream come true, building my own practice exactly how I wanted!

By May 1984 the Loughborough practice was up and running. A year later I was full time, quickly growing the practice and implementing the Health Cultivation philosophy. I had nurses trained as treatment coordinators and oral health promoters and the team won awards for practising prevention in the NHS.

Everything was going well at the practice until the end of the 80s, when the UK went into recession and interest rates rose to over 15%. My bank closed my account and required me to pay off my large overdraft in six weeks. This was a really dark time for me; I had a fantastic practice and staff but couldn't even afford to pay their wages. Fortunately, I managed to find a bank that would refinance my practice. However, it was on the condition that I started focusing more on the business and profitability of the practice.

I found myself at a crossroads. Do I become a 'drill, fill and bill' dentist – which many colleagues found to be very profitable – or do I stick to my values and work out how to offer Health Cultivation AND make a profit? I was not in dentistry just to make money, so I decided to hire a business coach to transform the practice using the Total Quality Management (TQM) approach. During this time, I earned nothing from the practice and relied on a small income as Programme Director for the Leicester VT scheme. This was a very stressful time; I had very little income and could barely pay the mortgage. This hardship did finally pay off, however. After two years we achieved ISO 9002 TQM accreditation and the business was turning over a profit.

The next big turning point came during the change in the NHS contract in the early 90s. I realised my philosophy of Health Cultivation could no longer be delivered under the new NHS contract and so, with much regret, I had to make the difficult decision to leave the NHS. At this time, I also took on a very talented Associate, Nilesh Shah, who I met through the VT scheme. Nilesh eventually became my business partner.

Nilesh also visited the Pankey Institute and we converted from NHS to a relationship-based private practice. We completed a large expansion and upgrade project in 2001 and the practice continued to grow and become more profitable. Nilesh provided the difficult dentistry (such as surgery and implants) and I did the simple stuff.

When I left the NHS I also gave up my VT Programme Director position. The experience inspired me to take a master's in Clinical Education and I became interested in practice-based research as a result. My TQM experience also led to teaching programmes for FDs on Clinical Governance and Audit. I have personally reviewed over 2000 audits in my career!

In 2006 I became Invisalign certified and fell in love with the system's ability to support comprehensive care. This led to a large increase in my adult orthodontic practice.

All was going well until the age of fifty, when I broke my arm and required nine weeks off clinical work. This was a good point in my life to reflect on my career. Soon my world was full of non-clinical work, including teaching, research in occlusion with Dr Ron Presswood and working with the FGDP. Since I was enjoying the non-clinical work so much, I made the decision to sell my share of the practice and work part time as an Associate

This new-found freedom allowed me to set up The Dental Business Academy, an online education company providing CPD and qualifications to the dental team. My teaching involvement with Invisalign also grew and recently, through Aligner Consulting, I have been delivering the Invisalign Go programme. Currently I am working with Dr Raman Aulakh on a post-graduate Diploma in Aligner Therapy.

What is success?

Success for me can be defined as feeling 'prosperous'. This means a level of financial security, of course, but also positive relationships with family, friends and at work.

Success is also overcoming major challenges and disasters in your life whilst still retaining your values.

Top tips for success

Dr Pankey said: "I never saw a tooth walk into my practice." My first job in every consultation is to build a relationship with my patient.

Your attitude will make the difference between success and failure, whenever you qualified. I have seen this in hundreds of young dentists I have worked with.

There is no such thing as a 'perfect' life – enjoy the journey, because you will never reach the point of perfection.

Cricketer to Dentist

Dr Monik Vasant
BChd MFGDP MSc

Dr Monik Vasant qualified from the University of Leeds in 2003. With a passion for minimal invasive dentistry, Monik has become a leading expert in this field, including mastering the use of composite techniques to produce beautiful smiles. He is the principal at two practices, Fresh Dental, in Bolton and London and works between both clinics. Monik is globally recognised in his field for lecturing internationally and running his own courses – Totally Composite (a two-day composite master class) and Totally Aesthetics (a year-long course in minimally invasive aesthetic dentistry).

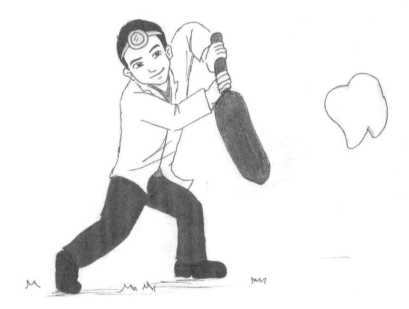

As a youngster, I was never interested in school. My main passion was cricket and I wanted to be a cricketer! I wasn't very studious and subsequently did not do well in my GCSE exams. I had some family members who I looked up to and respected who were dentists, so I always had a career in dentistry at the back of my mind.

My A-levels didn't begin very well either until I realised I wouldn't be able to make it as a cricketer, so I turned my attentions to getting into dentistry. However, my teachers told me I had no chance of becoming a dentist. Fuelled on by this, something inside me awoke! I started focusing on my studies and did well in my A-levels. Unfortunately, applications to dental schools were based on previous exam results and predicted A-level grades, none of which were great, leading to multiple rejections from the universities. Luckily, I did well in my A-level modules which meant good grades looked highly likely, so my headmaster wrote a letter to Leeds University – the only university that had not rejected me – and advised them that my predicted A-level grades were not correct. This paid off and I managed to secure a place.

My journey to get into university had been difficult, so whilst I was there I made sure I studied hard and made the most of the opportunity, including getting involved with sports and the dental society.

I qualified from university in 2003 and moved back home to Manchester for vocational training, which was a great experience and I learnt a lot. Following this, my plan was to move to London, but a great job opportunity came up in an NHS practice in Salford. I took it and stayed there for about four years. During this time, I became increasingly bored with the standard type of drill and fill dentistry and felt I had more to offer my patients; I did enjoy my composite work but had not completed any further training. I decided to start focusing on this and was recommended by a friend of mine to do a year course. I really enjoyed the programme and learnt lots. By now I was starting to think about becoming a practice owner. A friend I made on the course told me about an NHS tender available in the Bolton area so we decided to apply for this tender together. I spent a lot of time gathering detailed information for the tender application and also found a property in an ideal location to set up the practice. We had an offer accepted on the property before getting the NHS tender – but luckily we won it!

We then had the task of converting this property, which was at the time a house, into a three-surgery dental practice. The practice opened in 2008 and began doing really well; after a few years we even managed to expand to five surgeries. At this point my wife had to move to London for her work, and so I would work three or four long days at the Bolton practice and then spend some time down in London with her. On top of this I was also studying part time, a master's degree in restorative dentistry at the University of Manchester, which I completed in 2013. In the midst of all this I was asked to assist on various postgraduate restorative courses, which I enjoyed. However, I became more disillusioned with the traditional type of aggressive restorative dentistry and started to follow my passion for composite dentistry by travelling the world and learning from the masters, including people such as Newton Fahl, Didier Dietschi and Pascal Magne.

After my travels I was approached by Coltene to help run some MIRIS composite workshops, which was a great experience.

My next endeavour was to focus on opening a second practice, but this time in London. My uncle previously owned a small practice in Russell Square but had sold it to someone else. However, I heard this dentist was looking to sell the practice as he had moved away and it was struggling. I wanted to give it a go, so I purchased the practice in 2013. At the same time I bought out my wonderful business partner in Bolton. The Bolton practice continues to do well and has recently been extended to seven surgeries.

Slowly the practice in London has grown and currently I work one or two days in Bolton and two days in London. Growing the practice in London was by far the hardest thing I have had to do but with a lot of persistence we have managed it. Over time my clinical work has become more focused on minimally invasive aesthetics and restorative. I use Invisalign a lot to assist me in my restorative dentistry and this led to the company inviting me to be on their European Aesthetic Dentistry Advisory Board; more recently I've become head of the UK Invisalign Advisory Board and their UK GDP ambassador, which involves me teaching and lecturing at some of their courses and events.

After working with Coltene for several years, I really wanted to set up my own composite course, backed by the company. They would help with advertising and promoting the course, which would run all over the UK, three days spread over three weeks. We ran this course for two years but unfortunately there was little interest and it did not go well. Lecturing to only two or three people was soul destroying! I was about to give up on lecturing but I decided to give it one last shot and set up my own course, independent of company sponsorship, and condensed it down to a weekend programme in London. This was the game changer! The first course filled up to maximum capacity and I learnt that dentists don't like taking time off work; a weekend programme works better. Since then we have been running regular programmes to full houses, every two weeks. We have also taken the course internationally and have run programmes in the Middle East and Europe. More recently, we have launched a one-year programme on minimal invasive aesthetic dentistry. Teaching has truly been a rollercoaster ride, but I am very humbled at how well it has taken off.

I continue to have a passion for clinical work and enjoy the balance between teaching and clinical dentistry. To me it is very important to *do* what I teach and not just teach, as I can constantly learn and evolve in both the clinical and teaching environments. It also ensures that what I teach is current and relevant.

What is success?

Success is having inner content.

Top tips for success

Push yourself to be the best you can be.

Be persistent in achieving your goals.

Focus on your dentistry and good things will come.

Take time to master your profession; don't try to run before you can walk.

Whatever You Do, Do It Well

Dr Reena Wadia
BDS Hons (Lond) MJDF RCS (Eng) MClinDent (Perio) MPerio RCS (Edin)
FHEA

Dr Reena Wadia qualified from Bart's and The London in 2011. Following general practice and experience in the hospital setting, Reena completed a part-time speciality training programme in periodontology at Guy's Hospital. She now runs her own specialist referral practice, RW Perio, at Lister House, Wimpole Street.

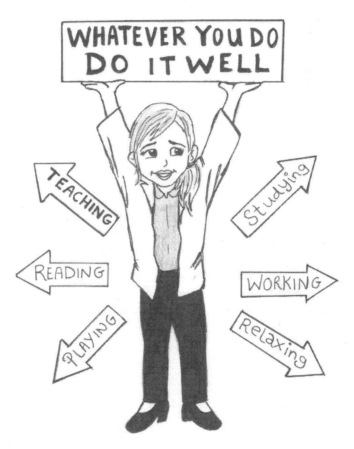

I'm 30. British Indian. Born, educated and live in London. I graduated from Bart's and The London in 2011. I completed my dental foundation training and had a fantastic year thanks to the team at MK Vasant & Associates. I was then lucky enough to be offered a Senior House Officer post at Guy's Hospital, where my time was equally split between the restorative and oral surgery departments. During this year, I kept my hand in practice by working in a general and specialist periodontal practice, before deciding to join the speciality training pathway.

I completed a part-time four-year speciality training programme in periodontology whilst working in practice. This was helpful as I could implement what I was learning on the course in practice. I spent a few years working with the Harley Street Dental Group and Woodford Dental Care before setting up my own clinic. I've always enjoyed hospital care as well as practice, so I am now also working one day a week as an associate specialist at King's College Dental Hospital.

I am passionate about education and was privileged enough to be a part-time clinical tutor for the undergraduate as well as the hygiene therapy students at Bart's and The London. I currently run regular courses for young dentists and hygienists, which I very much enjoy. I also like to share what I learn through my blog (www.reenawadia.com). As well as running my own blog I have also been given the opportunity to be the social media officer for the British Society of Periodontology and European Society of Periodontology.

I endeavour to contribute to the profession through my other positions, including board member of the Faculty of General Dental Practice, committee member of the British Dental Association, junior trustee of the Oral Dental & Dental Research Trust and co-editor for the British Dental Journal.

As much I love the wonderful world of teeth (and gums, of course), I have lots of other hobbies to keep me occupied! I enjoy keeping fit and I'm always up for a challenge. I'm also passionate about photography, making (and eating) desserts, travelling and spiritual development.

What is success?

Everyone's definition of success is different. For me it's doing what you want to be doing at all times!

I also quite like Tim Ferriss' definition of success; he explains, "it's a combination of achievement and appreciation. Achievement without appreciation makes you ambitious but miserable. Appreciation without achievement makes you unambitious but happy."

Top tips for success

Work out your WHY. What you are chasing? What is the ultimate outcome for you at the end of the day? Seems like an obvious question but it's often overlooked. I love this quote: "It's not how well you play the game, it's deciding what game you want to play."

Don't use the excuse: "I don't have time." Lack of time is actually lack of priorities. In the same way, focus on being productive instead of busy.

Tomorrow becomes never. No matter how small the task, take the first step now. If you feel overwhelmed, just focus on the next right step.

Be patient – nothing great happens overnight.

Don't keep comparing yourself to others. Focus on yourself, focus on your journey and don't measure success/progress using someone else's ruler.

Find a mentor – I feel blessed to have been surrounded by exceptionally inspirational dental professionals. Over time, a few of these individuals have become my mentors. By sharing their knowledge and experience, my mentors have become trusted advisors and role models. Their support and enthusiasm has encouraged me to reach my full potential and their advice has made a significant difference in my ability to successfully steer through the early years of my career. So find someone senior whose values and approach matches yours and they will be able to share the quickest way to achieve what you want.

'Everyone backs a winner' is the best piece of business advice I've received from one of my mentors, Asif Syed. Quite simply, the fastest route to success is to ask someone who knows. But successful people are busy, resulting in a catch 22 situation. However, if you work hard to successfully implement any advice they give you, they will always give you more. If you work harder to demonstrate progress, they will help you more as they believe you have the determination to succeed.

After which, assistance arrives in many forms. In contrast, I have rarely found these same inspiring individuals give up their valuable time to unlock this process to help someone who just asked for help as they are struggling.

Pay attention to the kinds of people you surround yourself with. Remember, you are the average of the five people you associate with most.

Make space for down time. This may mean saying "no" to less important invitations.

Always maintain integrity, no matter what. Integrity is the only path where you will never get lost.

The Story So Far!

Professor Nairn Wilson CBE
DSc(h.c.) FDS FFGDP FFD FKC

Professor Nairn Wilson graduated from the University of Edinburgh in 1973 and has made huge contributions in the field of dentistry. Throughout his illustrious career Nairn has achieved numerous honours and awards for his contribution to dentistry. Highlights of his career include former Professor of Restorative Dentistry and Dean and Head of the University of Manchester Dental School and King's College London, and former president of the GDC and the British Dental Association. His expertise encompasses the regulation of dentistry, international trends in dental education, tooth-coloured filling materials and related systems, and minimally invasive approaches to conservative dentistry.

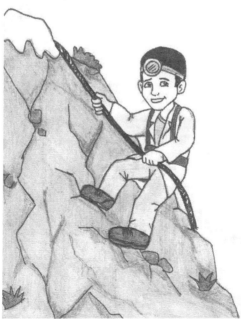

Following dalliances with careers in medicine and marine biology, I followed my father into dentistry. My five years as a dental student in Edinburgh were a good mix of hard work and play. During these formative years in my career I learnt the more I put into it, the more I got in return – a lesson which continues to serve me well to this day.

On graduation in 1973, I faced the difficulty of telling my father that I didn't know what I was going to do in dentistry, but I had decided that I was not going to join his practice. Considering some experience of hospital practice to be a good start to whatever I eventually decided to do, I accepted the offer of a House Officer position at Edinburgh Dental Hospital. Within months, I was asked if I would consider a temporary lecturer post to provide sabbatical leave cover. Given the prospect of a substantial pay increase (£850 to £1500 per annum), I accepted, not appreciating that this would be the beginning of my career in clinical academic dentistry. The individual who took sabbatical leave quickly decided that he was not going to return, and I was encouraged to apply for the vacant lectureship which offered another £300 in annual salary. So, it could be said that I was lured into academia by money; however, I enjoyed teaching and research and did not take much persuading to go for the lectureship.

A year or so into my lectureship in Restorative Dentistry at Edinburgh, I was head-hunted to take up a lectureship in Conservative Dentistry in Manchester, with the prospect of being able to immediately register for a MSc by research. I anticipated the move to Manchester being for a few years only. Little did I know that it would be for the next 27 years, culminating in me becoming a Pro-Vice Chancellor of the university, after having been Dean of the Dental School.

Three years into my initial position in Manchester, I found myself seconded to what became ICI Dental to work on novel dental biomaterials. I became the lead clinician on the project to develop and introduce visible light-cured systems into dentistry. The first visible light-cured material was Fotofil – the first single paste composite, accompanied by the Fotofil visible light quartz halogen curing unit – another first in dentistry, produced by ICI and marketed by Johnson & Johnson. Occlusin, the first visible light-cured composite for the restoration of posterior teeth, followed quickly thereafter, together with the Luxor curing light, marketed by the then newly formed ICI Dental. Other products, including Opalux – the first multi-purpose (anterior or posterior)/ multi-shade visible light-cured composite system; Tripton – a smear layer mediated dentine bonding system; and Epitex finishing strip system, which remains popular to this day. These were very exciting times. I travelled the world, was involved in lots of cutting edge research, much of which could not be published for commercial reasons, and developed an international network of colleagues, many of whom I undertook collaborative research with in years to come.

When ICI Dental, including Coe Laboratories, acquired on the way, was bought out by the GC Corporation, I returned to full time academia, with the good fortune to be appointed Professor of Conservative in Manchester at 36 years of age, within months of my secondment having come to an end. Before becoming Dean in Manchester in 1992, my Chair had become the first Chair in Restorative in the UK and I was heavily involved in many different organisations home and abroad, including the Faculty of Dental Surgery of the Royal College of Surgeons of Edinburgh, which I was Dean of between 1995 and 1998 – another fantastic experience with lots of international commitments.

My career then took another quite unexpected turn in 1999 when I was elected President of the old, self-regulation style, 52-member strong General Dental Council (GDC). This was a career-changing development, but with the downside that there would be no going back to my Pro-Vice Chancellor position in Manchester. In anticipation of having to seek a position overseas – North America, the Far East or Australasia – following the end of my term as President of the GDC, I spent all my holidays while President of the GDC being a Visiting Professor in various places around the world, including the University of Florida, where I spent several summers accompanied by my family.

Near the end of my time at the GDC, the position of Dean and Head of King's College London Dental Institute (KCLDI) became vacant. To cut a long story short, I spent 12-18 months being both President of the GDC and Dean and Head of KCLDI – 80 hours of intense, challenging work a week, on a good week!

My 11+ years as Dean and Head of KCLDI was another exceptional phase of my career; one of the best, if not the best job in clinical academic dentistry in the world. Thanks to the support extended to me by the world class staff of KCLDI, I remained research active and was able to continue to write and publish throughout my time at King's. Regrettably, the many different calls on my time, especially when I became Deputy Vice Principal for Health at King's in 2009, took me away from clinical practice, which I had always enjoyed, having served as an Honorary Consultant in Restorative Dentistry since 1982.

Following my retirement from King's in 2012, I have had the good fortune to work in many different areas, with the presidency of the British Dental Association being a highlight of the last few years – yet another truly memorable experience. This, together with having time and opportunity to do such things as support dental charities as a Patron or Trustee, and spend time writing and publishing on the history and future of dentistry, gives me lots to do and think about.

Now, I am delighted to be heading up the initiative to form what is hoped will become a Royal College for Dentistry – a final piece in the jigsaw of dentistry becoming a fully recognised and established profession. What better way to celebrate 50 years since entering dental school than to found a College for Dentistry?

Reading the above, the impression may be gained that it has been 'all work and no play'. While my work/life balance could never have been described as good, I have had, or made time to do many things outside dentistry, but that's a story for another day.

I am indebted to my family, especially my wife, Margaret, formerly Consultant in Restorative Dentistry and Clinical Director, University Dental Hospital of Manchester and now, amongst other positions, Honorary Curator of the BDA Museum and Editor of the Dental Historian, without whom much of what I have done would not have been possible.

I must pay tribute also to all those who have helped and supported me throughout my career; many achievements credited to me were a tremendous team effort.

Where next? Watch this space!

What is success?

Making a lasting difference, with clear sight of the next challenge.

Top tips for success

Keep well informed, have vision and determination, and seek to realise your potential.

About the Authors

Dream It, Do It

Nafisa Mughal
Dip Dent Hyg RCS (Eng)

Nafisa Mughal is the co-author of this book. She is a dental hygienist and qualified from the Eastman Dental Hospital in 2008. She has a passion for facial aesthetics and has her own aesthetic business. She also writes articles in Dental Health and Oral Health journals for hygienists and provides training on facial aesthetics. She is a keen advocate for empowering hygienists/therapists to reach their full potential.

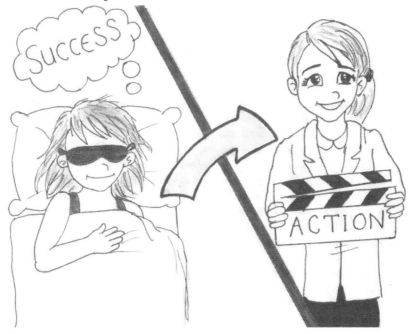

Growing up, I had no one around me that was in the dental or medical profession. My grandparents immigrated to East London in the 60s and worked in factories, restaurants and other types of labour intensive work. This 'hard work' mentality was instilled in my father, who owned his own business.

My first memory of considering a career within dentistry was when we were selecting our work experience placements. I decided to go for a placement at a local dental surgery. Back then there were not these fancy studios with high tech equipment, just a tired-looking rundown two-surgery practice that had that 'dentist smell'.

I wasn't blown away by it, I have to say. Filing, making coffee and generally just hanging around didn't fill me with joy but I got through the two weeks knowing one thing for sure: I didn't want to be a dentist!

A few years passed and after I did my A-Levels I was at a bit of a loss as to what to do next. I found a place that looked interesting called the Eastman Dental Hospital. I browsed their website and came across the dental hygiene section and remember thinking, "That looks fun – and they earn decent money too!" I filled in the application form but later realised that the deadline for submitting had already passed. "Never mind," I thought, "I'll apply to do dental nursing and then apply for the following intake for hygiene."

I was accepted into the dental nursing training school and honestly, I hated it! That was until I had my rotation in the periodontology department. Oh my goodness! I had found something that really interested me. I was much more than a dental nurse up in that periodontal department. I was a sponge, learning all about bacteria and plaque and the pitfalls of not flossing properly! I wanted to be on the other side of the dental chair, educating the patient and helping them achieve great oral health. That's when I sent off my application for dental hygiene and was invited for an interview a few weeks later.

I was about halfway through my dental nursing training when I received a call from the principal of the dental hygiene school within Eastman Dental Hospital. She asked me a few questions, then offered me a place on the course. I felt like I was floating. I remember telling her that I was still in training for dental nursing but that would be okay since I'd only started it to gain some experience while I waited for the dental hygiene intake to open again. To my horror, the principal decided I should defer to the following year so I could complete my dental nurse training. I had no choice but to agree to this and continued to study dental nursing knowing that I would be coming back to study dental hygiene. After that though, dental nursing didn't seem so bad.

I qualified as a dental hygienist in 2008 and was out in the big wide world.

I loved working in central London and the buzz of the city carried me into work in the mornings. I never used to get the Monday blues and my friends thought I was mad because I looked at dirty teeth all day and loved it! It wasn't the dirty teeth I loved; it was providing that education and motivation to the patients and then seeing the difference in their oral health once they applied the things we talked about at their appointments. I felt like I was making a difference.

I did want something else though. I wanted to work on Harley Street.

My husband attended a training course and mentioned to one of the other dentists on the course that I was a hygienist. As it happened, he was looking for a hygienist for his practice. I was invited for an interview and when I looked up the practice I found that it was on Harley Street! I was offered the job and achieved my goal.

We had moved out of London so sadly I didn't stay at that practice for too long as eventually the horror of commuting by train from Bedfordshire started to take its toll.

After a year of loving dental hygiene, I decided I wanted to do more, so I trained in tooth whitening. I started to notice that patients loved coming in to see me even more when they knew they were having something cosmetic as opposed to standard hygiene treatment. I loved that they looked forward to their appointment and decided to train in administering Botulinum Toxin so I could help more patients feel good.

I got the bug for aesthetics. I loved seeing a difference in my patients' confidence and that spurred me on to train in dermal fillers and other skin rejuvenating treatments. I also completed a diploma in semi-permanent makeup techniques to add to my aesthetics treatments.

For a few years I was comfortably plodding along in practice, only offering aesthetics to patients who enquired about it. It wasn't until I went to an aesthetic medicine conference that I realised my passion is helping people look and feel good through aesthetics. I made a decision that day that I was going to set up my own aesthetics practice and slowly reduce the days that I did dental hygiene.

In under a year, I set up my own aesthetics company and increased the amount of aesthetics I was offering over 100%.

I felt that I needed to share this with other hygienists, so I contacted the editors of Oral Health magazine and Dental Health Journal and asked if I could write some articles for them about hygienists offering facial aesthetics, as it seemed to be a bit of a grey area. They both replied with a resounding yes and I got to follow another passion of mine, writing.

I am still loving offering aesthetics and am currently running training programmes to offer aesthetics training to other hygienists and therapists.

I found that my greatest passion in life is empowering others, be that through helping them achieve great oral health, boosting their confidence in the way they look, or teaching them a new skill and helping them implement it.

What is success?

Success to me is achieving your goals and dreams, irrespective of other people's opinions. If your main goal in life is to be working in the best practice in your town, and you're there, you are successful. Or if you always wanted to be a hygienist and you have trained and qualified, you are a success! Success should only be measured by your standards, not by anyone else's.

Top tips for success

My top tip for success is do what you love to do. Don't be afraid to dream. Push forward and don't let anyone or anything limit you in achieving what it is that you set out to do, and not listen to people who bring you down or don't encourage you to follow your passion. If this is the case, hang around with other people, those who raise you up rather than bring you down.

Never Give Up!

Dr Shakir Mughal
BDS (Hons)

Dr Shakir Mughal qualified in 2005 from King's College London. Soon after, he began a journey of postgraduate training leading him to courses all over the UK, Europe and USA, including The Pankey Institute in Miami. Shakir has a special interest in orthodontics and is a co-owner of two dental practices in Hertfordshire and Buckinghamshire. He also has a passion for human behaviour, mindset and psychology, leading him to become a student of Neuro-Linguistic Programming (NLP).

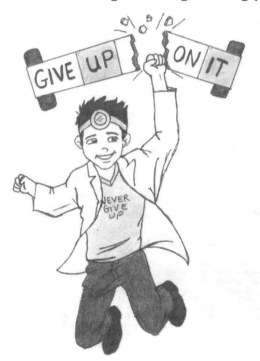

'Never give up' is the mantra I have always lived by; from losing five stones to running five marathons, I never gave up! I was born in Kenya and moved over to the UK at the age of one, after my father suddenly passed away. My mother came to the UK to give our family a better chance of success. At an early age the 'never give up' philosophy was instilled in me by my mother, who had been through so much.

At school I was below average in intelligence but made up for it in hard work and determination. My mother taught me the importance of education and at the age of 13 I managed to get a scholarship to a private school, after three failed attempts. I never gave up as I knew I needed the best possible education to succeed.

As a keen lover of art and science I decided I would combine the two and apply to study dentistry. Following several rejections from universities, I finally landed a place at King's College London.

At university, I had some of the best times of my life and loved London life. After five great years of both working hard and playing hard, I managed to qualify with honours in 2005.

Following university, I struggled to find vocational training (VT) but after several rejections, I managed to secure a VT position in Bedfordshire. I loved my VT year and enjoyed the mix of clinical work and the study days. However, I quickly realised that I did not want to do general dentistry forever, particularly amalgam fillings! Equally, I did not want to specialise and so decided to begin a postgraduate training journey which to this day I am still on.

I was lucky in that down the road from my VT practice was Dr Raj Ahlowalia, who opened my eyes to a completely new level of dentistry. Spurred on by him, I decided to travel to Miami to study at the Pankey Institute, which gave me a new level of confidence in dealing with patients and also providing more comprehensive dentistry.

Following my VT year, I stayed on at the practice but eventually decided to leave to work in other more cosmetic-focused private practices. Over the years I gained lots of experience working in a variety of predominantly private practices in Hertfordshire, Birmingham and Milton Keynes whilst still attending countless courses and study clubs.

As the years went on and the type of dentistry I was delivering became more complex, I began to question how aggressive my techniques were in terms of drilling teeth and I decided to learn some simple short-term orthodontics. From these initial courses I soon began to realise I had a great passion and affinity for orthodontics and began focusing on this more in my practices. Over the years I have steadily increased this part of my practice and have continued studying so I can take on more advanced cases.

In 2011 I then took the plunge into co-buying my first practice with my old university roommate! Practice number two was purchased in 2014 with my wife.

Becoming a principal was certainly a big shock and to this day continues to be a challenging but rewarding role. Nothing had prepared me to run a business and balancing the clinical and non-clinical work was a massive test.

Since becoming a principal and facing the challenges of being a business owner I have turned to reading and I've studied human behaviour, psychology, mindset and how to be successful in life. This has taken me on an incredible, life-changing journey and continues to do so.

Currently I divide my time between practices, providing general dentistry, private orthodontics and spending one day a week focusing on the business side and how to grow both practices. When I am not at the practices my focus turns to my new-found passion for studying and reading about success.

What is success?

For me, success is about progress, which equals happiness. Progress is a need to fulfil a constant hunger. A hunger to learn, a hunger to grow, a hunger to serve and a hunger to give.

Top tips for success

This is a hard one; I think I could write a whole book on just this topic alone! Here are a few of my more important tips:

Take 100% responsibility for yourself. No excuses, no blame; you are the master of your own fate!

Create your own vision and goals and know exactly what you want.

Know WHY you want it.

Take action to go and get it.

Above all, NEVER GIVE UP!

The Secret to Dental Success

Wow, what a collection of stories! We hope you agree and also hope you have taken something away from each and every story that you have read. We truly hope these stories and tips will inspire you in your life, not just in dentistry but also outside in the big wide world!

'The history of the world is but the biography of great individuals.'
Thomas Carlyle

All our experts differ in their backgrounds and upbringings but share the same motivation and desire to succeed. What success means to them is different, as you have seen through their own definitions of success. Interestingly, their top tips have shown many commonalities and in this final chapter we have taken all the top tips from the experts and divided them into dental-specific tips and life tips to create the ultimate set of success principles for you. We hope you will begin to follow these principles and over time see your life transformed.

Success in Dentistry

For success within dentistry you must accept you are a professional. That means many things but primarily, focusing on your patients, putting them at the centre of everything you do, discovering their needs and wants and then addressing them. Sometimes it means doing it when you don't want to. Dentistry is not an easy career, but you are fortunate to be able to do it. You must respect and earn the trust that people put in you.

Do as much learning while you can and never stop learning. Getting your BDS is only the start. Once you stop learning, stop being curious, stop developing yourself, stop looking beyond where you are, you are going backwards. Remember the more you learn, the more you earn!

'If I am through learning, I am through.'
John Wooden

Dentistry can be a very rewarding career but also at times very stressful. Ensure you look after yourself and your wellbeing, both physically and mentally.

Always remember our profession is here to serve and help people. If you stick to this principle the success will come.

'From my first days as an entrepreneur, I've felt the only mission worth pursuing in business is to make people's lives better.'
Richard Branson

Find a mentor. By sharing their knowledge and experience, mentors become trusted advisors and role models. Find someone senior whose values and approach matches yours and they will be able to share the quickest way to achieve what you want.

'Success leaves clues.'
Tony Robbins

Find your niche in the dental world, as this gives you your unique selling point. Companies need a unique selling point but so do individuals. If you do exactly what everyone else does you won't stand out from the crowd.

'The whole secret to a successful life is to find out what is one's destiny to do, and then to do it.'
Henry Ford

Love your patients and love your team.

Build trust between yourself and the patient by having empathy, being honest, and developing great communication skills – including learning the art of conversation. Create time to talk to patients and communicate with them to provide patient-centred care.

'I never saw a tooth walk into my practice.'
Dr Pankey

Just follow the Golden Rule and treat people how you would want to be treated yourself.

Photograph all your cases – or you are missing out on the biggest learning experience in dentistry.

Success doesn't happen overnight. It takes time. Be patient and listen. Listen to your mentors, your peers but most importantly, your patients.

'Our greatest weakness lies in giving up. The most certain way to succeed is always to try one more time.'
Thomas A Edison

Take time to master your profession; don't try to run before you can walk.

'Stop chasing the money and start chasing the passion.'
Tony Hsieh

Try to find an environment to work in where you are happy and be a part of perpetuating that happy environment too.

Have a good work / life balance; we work to live, we don't live to work. Leave work at work and enjoy yourself!

Time management is critical for success; you must balance your time of working in the business and on the business.

Some of the comments and feedback on social media can be very negative and critical; our advice is to not take any of these comments seriously. Don't get distracted or be made to feel inferior by the antics of some on social media. Keep your head down, get your work done, get the experience and be the best you can.

'Too many people spend money they haven't earned to buy things they don't want to impress people they don't like.'
Will Rogers

Success in Life

Create your own vision and goals. Know exactly what you want.

'You control your future, your destiny. What you think about comes about. By recording your dreams and goals on paper, you set in motion the process of becoming the person you most want to be. Put your future in good hands – your own.'
Mark Victor Hansen

Work out your WHY. What are you chasing? What is the ultimate outcome for you at the end of the day?

'The two most important days in your life are the day you were born and the day you find out why.'
Mark Twain

Take 100% responsibility for yourself. No excuses, no blame; you are the master of your own fate!

'I attribute success to this: I never gave or took any excuse.'
Florence Nightingale

Take action and go and get it.

'Inaction breeds doubt and fear. Action breeds confidence and courage. If you want to conquer fear, do not sit at home and think about it. Go out and get it.'
Dale Carnegie

Do what you love to do. Don't be afraid to dream. Push forward and don't let anyone or anything limit you in achieving what it is that you set out to do, and not listen to people who bring you down or don't encourage you to follow your passion. If this is the case, hang around with other people, those who raise you up rather than bring you down.

> *'All our dreams can come true if we have the courage to pursue them.'*
> **Walt Disney**

Push yourself to be the best you can be.

> *'Don't wish it were easier, wish you were better.'*
> **Jim Rohn**

Do something you enjoy. Find your passion and the rest will follow.

> *'Success is no accident. It is hard work, perseverance, learning, studying, sacrifice and most of all, love of what you are doing and learning to do.'*
> **Pele**

Focus on what you are good at and become a master at that.

> *'Your true success in life begins only when you make the commitment to become excellent at what you do.'*
> **Brian Tracy**

Be persistent in achieving your goals.

> *'The greatest danger for most of us is not that our aim is too high and we miss it, but that it is too low and we reach it.'*
> **Michelangelo**

You have to work really, *really* hard to succeed and don't dabble. If you wish to succeed then you must immerse yourself in your goals and live them.

'Talent is cheaper than table salt. What separates the talented individual from the successful one is a lot of hard work.'
Stephen King

Always have your foot on the accelerator and keep moving forward.

'Nothing is in the way, everything is on the way.'
John Di Martini

Don't keep comparing yourself to others. Focus on yourself, focus on your journey and don't measure success/progress using someone else's ruler.

'It's time to start living the life you imagined.'
Henry James

Be a people person and build relationships with people.

Have excellent communication and listening skills.

There is no such thing as failure, only feedback.

'Our greatest glory is not in never falling, but in rising every time we fall.'
Confucius

There is not always a wrong or right, as long as you are confident in yourself that you are doing the right thing.

Don't use the excuse: "I don't have time." Lack of time is actually lack of priorities. In the same way, focus on being productive instead of busy.

'You will never find time for anything. If you want time, you must make it.'
Charles Buxton

Tomorrow becomes never. No matter how small the task, take the first step now. If you feel overwhelmed, just focus on the next right step.

'Action is the foundational key to all success.'
Pablo Picasso

Make space for down time. This may mean saying "no" to less important invitations.

Always maintain integrity, no matter what. Integrity is the only path where you will never get lost.

'Man is what he believes.'
Anton Chekhov

Know your strengths and your weaknesses and focus on improving upon your weaknesses, to at least neutralise, then develop them. Remember almost everything started as a weakness!

'You must take personal responsibility. You cannot change the circumstances, the seasons, or the wind, but you can change yourself.'
Jim Rohn

Invest in assets that will produce passive income every month, no matter what you do yourself.

And above all ... NEVER GIVE UP!!

We hope you enjoyed those tips and, more importantly, we hope you will try to apply them. Knowledge is not enough. You need to take action as well! Try to make these tips part of your daily routine and they will slowly become part of your routine habits, just like brushing your teeth. These habits will eventually lead you on to great things.

One important point to finish on is realising that success does not equal wealth or money. This book is not intended to make you more money. As you have read the stories, you may or may not have noticed that none of our experts linked success solely to money. Everyone's definition of success is different. The most important thing is to define your own success and then go out and get it!

Finally, we hope you will create your own dental success story!

'It's time to start living the life you've imagined.'
Henry James

Acknowledgements

A big thanks to all twenty-five experts featured in our book; your time, generosity and honesty with your stories has been truly inspiring to us.

A special thanks to Dr Harry Singh, who has helped us with the whole process of writing this book, and Seb Evans from FMC publications, who has helped with getting this project started.

Another big thank you to Dr Ash Parmar, who has kindly allowed us to support a charity he is currently the chairman of: Food for Life Vrindavan. Please visit www.fflv.org, for further information regarding this amazing charity. A proportion of the profit from every book sold will go to this charity.

We would also like to give a special big thank you to Kate Boakes, who skilfully produced all the illustrations.

Big thanks to all our friends, family members and dental colleagues who have supported this project.

35443079R00079

Printed in Great Britain
by Amazon